TECHNOMIC
PUBLISHING CO., INC.

THE VIEW FROM THE GURNEY UP

Dealing With People In
Crisis and Emergency

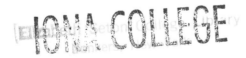
ARTHUR R. CIANCUTTI, M.D.

©TECHNOMIC Publishing Co., Inc. 1984
851 New Holland Avenue
Box 3535
Lancaster, Pennsylvania 17604

Printed in U.S.A.
Library of Congress Card No. 83-51731
ISBN 87762-338-4

"For Michelle"

TABLE OF CONTENTS

PREFACE

The chances are that, as a person trying to help other people in crisis, you derive enormous satisfaction from a sense that you are doing a good job. When you personally feel that you are doing a good job, it is partly because of your willingness to improve. Within the health care profession itself, the collective willingness to improve is demonstrated in the myriad of technological advances and new information that we are constantly weaving into the health care we provide.

This is not a book about technological advances or about developing a new formalized system of health care delivery. It is, rather, a book concerning the most important element in the successful delivery of help: your ability to care for and to communicate with patients and the other members of your team. Regardless of technological breakthroughs and changes in the formalized system of care delivery, all of us can more fully apply our competence to realize the ultimate goal of patient well-being. That is what this book is about.

Teamwork. . . Who, in all your training, really outlined the elements of teamwork and practically demonstrated its function?

Confusion. . . How many times a day to you experience it, great or small? Yet, were you actually trained to understand confusion and eliminate it?

Help. . . Do you ever try to help and wonder if you actually might be hindering?

Stress. . . Is it really inevitable?

This book, and particularly this expanded edition, is meant as a contribution to anyone who is dealing with another person or persons who are experiencing a crisis. Much of the language concerns crises of health, but the principles and intent, I believe, apply to anyone experiencing change or crisis in any arena of his or her life.

Arthur R. Ciancutti, M.D.

THE VIEW FROM THE GURNEY UP

The View From the Gurney Up

IMAGINE IT: YOU ARE THE PATIENT LYING FLAT ON YOUR BACK looking up. What do you see? Your environment is sterile and white glaring. The people looking down at you are strangers who are charged with the responsibility of helping you solve a problem you know nothing about. You, yourself, have the problem and no one else. While you are the star of the drama, you don't know your lines, and there's no rehearsal. The setting is frightening. Somewhere in the back of your mind a though lurks: at any moment some incredible horror may be wheeled past you, maybe even become a roommate, and you're a captive audience. And that is over and above your own problem.

No matter what that problem is, how minor or how major, you don't understand it and you think the problem is, at least, potentially dangerous, or you wouldn't be looking for help in the first place.

This is the viewpoint of the patient that we, as health care deliverers, deal with many times every day. Our ability to elicit trust in this situation is as important as knowing how to get a line in right now. Our ability to communicate, naturally, an understandable and tailormade solution to the patient's problem is as important as the solution itself. Effecting this natural communication is simple. It starts with an objective understanding of the patient's point of view. The most dramatic case, of course, is the patient presenting with an "emergency," but the principles apply to any situation that includes someone seeking help with a problem of health.

What is an emergency patient? First and foremost, he is a person who is waiting. He thinks he is in danger. He is in the midst of a dramatic experience over which he has, seemingly, little or no control. He is probably a little suspicious about emergency or health care settings to begin with. His immediate future is uncertain; maybe his whole future seems to him uncertain. He is disori-

1

ented to his immediate past in that his objective memory of the illness or injury event itself is blurred. His family or friends are worried and probably fussing about it. He may be in physical pain. He knows the care he receives is going to cost him for sure, whether it works or not. All of his uncertainties and fears are at play—about aging, about his career, about his family situation, and about the ways he has been using his life so far. He is surrounded by cold paraphernalia and mysterious compartments. He is probably embarassed already and is at least anticipating some possibly embarrassing procedure or question. He feels a little foolish just for getting sick or hurt in the first place. And through all of this high drama, the patient feels out of control. There is absolutely nothing he can do to solve the problem on his own.

Then you walk in.

Your first job, as all of ours always is in health care, is to begin stabilizing all aspects of the situation, including the body aspects of the situation, but also including the mind and emotional parts—the "human" elements. Dealing with the human part of the situation can be done effortlessly and in perfect harmony with your skills for dealing with the physical parts, once you actually intend to tune in to the whole situation.

Realize that this emergency or this health care problem is the patient's, not yours. He is the star; you are a vital part of the supporting cast. You are volunteering to assume *temporary,* albeit sometimes awesome, responsibility for a problem that is not yours. Since the problem is his and not yours, you do not have to be in an emergency yourself. When the staff—essentially strangers who are there to offer help—is flustered and confused, that attitude communicates to the patient. The effect, then, is to increase the instability in the situation, rather than to begin the stabilization process. Knowing yourself and remembering that the problem is the patient's and not yours adds to your armament in providing the kind of help that is going to work. You can then approach the patient calmly and with assurance, thereby being an example of stability yourself. This puts you in an ideal position to introduce yourself by name and function. "Hi, I'm Ms. Jones, I'm here to take your blood pressure, to examine you," or whatever is appropriate. This establishes *purpose.* Then ask something like, "Is that ok?", thereby eliciting the patient's *willingness* to have you help in certain ways with his problem. The patient, someone who is waiting, who feels in danger, and who feels out of control, now has been given a choice—the very first step for him in re-establishing control.

You now have begun to help the patient establish an island of stability amidst drama. No matter what your function on the health care team, be it of physician, nurse, aide, technician, ambulance attendant, peace officer, family member, or friend, you have just become a leader in this heretofore leaderless situation. The most effective way to lead in any situation, including this one, is to lead by example. Among your other skills and abilities, you can be a model of communication and of stability. This helps focus the patient's attention on the solution, on health or recovery, rather than just on the problem.

T   W   O

Whose Problem Is It?

A child is struck by a speeding auto.
A concert pianist cuts his finger.
A corporation executive suffers a cardiac arrest.
A photographer is hit in the eye.
A pregnant woman falls down a flight of stairs.

EACH OF THESE CASES IS AN EMERGENCY, SOMETIMES FOR only one person, sometimes for others as well. It is extremely important for those of us involved in emergency medical care to know with *whose* emergency we are dealing.

Every emergency involves danger and the potential of *serious personal loss.* The dangerous elements in each emergency are particular to the circumstances surrounding each individual event.

Danger is relative. It is a value assigned by humans to particular situations, and so it has no objective reality. Most people place a high value on life, so to most, the potential of death is considered the greatest of all dangers. A concert pianist, however, might well place the highest value on his ability to interpret and create music. He might consider a cut finger, involving the potential loss of this ability and a lifetime of musical inactivity, to be the greatest of all dangers.

To determine *whose* emergency is involved, each event should be considered in the light of our definition: An emergency involves danger and the potential of *serious personal loss.*

A child is struck by a speeding auto—Whose emergency? Primarily that of the child, of course, who is in danger of experiencing what most people consider the most serious personal loss—life. But this circumstance also is an emergency for the child's parents. They, too, face the dangerous potential of serious personal loss—the companionship of their child. The status of

5

emergency may even be assigned to the driver of the car because he, too, faces the potential of serious personal loss—his driver's license, his reputation, perhaps even his freedom. The emergency does not extend, however, to the child's playmates. Even if the child should die, their loss might be personal, but it would not be *serious*; they would find another playmate.

A concert pianist cuts his finger. Depending on his value system, as noted, this might be a very serious emergency indeed, even approaching the type involving loss of life. It might also be *serious* for music lovers and concert managers throughout the world, but for them it would not qualify as an emergency because it would not be *personal*.

A corporation executive suffers a cardiac arrest. For this executive, of course, this is an emergency with the dangerous potential of serious personal loss, possible loss of income, perhaps loss of life. The event also qualifies as an emergency for the man's immediate family, since there is the potential loss of a loved one. The corporation might find itself in a crisis, faced with production or personnel problems, but the crisis would be temporary and so not terribly *serious*. And since corporations, by definition, are impersonal entities, this event could have no *personal* effect on the company. The corporate employer would not be involved in the emergency.

A photographer is hit in the eye. If it's the eye the man puts to his camera, the man has an emergency involving danger and the potential of serious personal loss. His clients, however, face no emergency. They may be his personal friends and experience the potential loss on that score, but the possible loss of the photographer's services would not be *serious*. Other photographers are always available for assignments.

A pregnant woman falls down a flight of stairs. The definition of emergency certainly applies in this case to the woman, her husband, and perhaps to her unborn child. But the shoe repairman who did a bad job of putting new heels on her shoes experiences no emergency at all. Since he is involved in no *danger*, fears no potential *personal* loss, and probably is so unaware of his role in the event, he takes it no more *seriously* than he would any other accident reported in the newspaper.

It is of the utmost importance for those of us involved in emergency medical care to recognize that *we are not involved in the emergency itself*. We are not in danger. We do not suffer the potential of serious personal loss. Whose emergency? *It is not ours*.

If the emergency is not ours, why are we there? To solve problems, to change or stem the tide of events, to prevent unnecessary loss.

Each emergency poses a problem which requires immediate and purposeful action in order to achieve a solution. This is why we are there: to recognize the problem; to take decisive action to solve the problem; and to *meet, minimize, or eliminate the danger* and, by eliminating the danger, to eliminate the emergency.

Each of us must remember that we are in health care by choice. The emergencies themselves are not ours. The problems posed by the emergencies, however, *are* ours, and we have chosen to accept at least temporary responsibility for their quick and accurate solutions.

Adopting this objective stance will go a long way toward increasing our effectiveness when confronted with emergencies. We cannot afford to be less than objective. We cannot afford to pause in sorrow over the torn body of a little girl hit by a speeding automobile. To pause is to hesitate, and hesitation very often might prove fatal.

The same logic exactly applies to all health care problems brought to us for help. If we are to be compassionate and effective, we must recognize that our purpose is to provide help to somebody else to solve their problem, not ours. We cannot provide help as long as we are, to any degree, taking on someone else's problem as if it were our own. The ownership of the problem must be crystal clear. The patient has the health problem, and you have the problem of providing effective help to the patient for his health problem.

Help!

FEW AREAS IN HEALTH CARE ARE AS HIGHLY CHARGED, EMO-tionally, as the basic area of help.

Help is an action or inaction which enhances another person's well-being. It definitely is not the rescue of victims.

Help is not inherent in the world. It is not an entity or substance that can be found in our environment. It eludes all of the physical senses; still we know it is there when it occurs. Help is a transaction between people created by those people.

But what constitutes real help? Why are some people offended when we try to help them? Why is it difficult for some to accept help? Why is it difficult for others to give it? Why are our feelings hurt when we try to help and apparently fail?

Help is always a two-way street. Sometimes it is a multiple-laned freeway, but the traffic always flows in two directions. Every successful transaction of help involves at least one helper and one person receiving help. Each must score on several points for the help transaction to be successful.

What is required of the person receiving help for the transaction to be successful?

(1) He must be willing to receive help. Attempts to force help on someone who does not want it will meet with resistance and cause frustration. The only way to help a person who is unwilling to receive help is to leave him alone.

(2) He must have defined a specific need or desire for help. The more precisely a person receiving help knows what kind of help he needs, the more likely he will get what he actually wants. It is not at all necessary that he need help. He may simply desire help with something which, actually, he could accomplish by himself.

(3) He must be willing and able to ask for help, and he must communicate the specific need or desire. The more directly he asks

for exactly what he wants, the more likely he is to get what he wants. Indirect or silent dramatizations requesting help usually result in indirect or inaccurate efforts to help and more frustrations on both sides.

Many people are unwilling to ask for help. They are not willing to make their needs or desires known. This involves communication that is sometimes embarrassing. Others ask for help indirectly or even silently, dramatizing their thought that, "if he *really* loved me, he would *know* what I want." This is an interesting exercise, but it is seldom efficient in obtaining real help of any kind.

(4) He must find someone who is willing and able to provide the help. The two-way flow of the help transaction presupposes a giver as well as a receiver of the help. My own experience is that each of us is almost continually surrounded by people who are willing and able helpers but who remain hidden from us because they are not sought out.

(5) The person receiving help can acknowledge or thank the helper. A verbal or material acknowledgment completes the help cycle on the receiver's side of the transaction and usually increases the chances that he will receive more of what he wants from the helper in future transactions.

And what does a successful help transaction demand of the helper?

(1) The helper, of course, must be willing to help. More important, he genuinely must be willing to provide the kind of help being requested. In other words, he must be willing to abandon his own ideas and standards of what might be "best" for the person requesting help—and simply provide what is stated as wanted.

(2) He must be able to help. That is, he must have the time and ability to provide the kind of help being requested.

(3) The helper must be in contact with the person seeking help. He must know someone who wants to receive the kind of help he is willing to supply.

(4) The helper must be willing to receive acknowledgment or thanks from the person he has helped.

(5) He must be able to experience and communicate his own appreciation for the opportunity to help. This expression completes the help transaction.

Failure on any of the ten points listed above results in a failure of the help transaction.

Failure on any of the ten points not only produces frustration but often is fraught with dangers.

When we, as medical helpers, try to force on someone a kind of help that is not wanted, we meet either outright resistance or pretended acceptance. The end result is a sense of incompletion on both sides.

A person who tries to force help on another usually is trying to advertise his willingness to help. Actually, he wants to be noticed more than he wants to help. In the health field, we frequently encounter the problems of too much help being offered by ourselves or others. People, especially patients, often experience a real lift and a measure of personal success if they are permitted to help themselves. Even if it appears to us, as potential helpers, that a person needs help, it often is the best course to stay away completely or to back off and await developments, meanwhile expressing our willingness to help if we are asked. *It is actively helping to leave someone alone who doesn't want help.*

We must recognize that rescuing is not helping. Although habitual rescuers are people with good intentions, rescuing usually causes frustration and resentment. Nearly all rescuers conceive of themselves as being "nice" to the "poor victims." This attitude places the helper above the person helped and denies the truth of equality between people. This hardly is conducive to the give-and-take of a true help situation. This attitude, in fact, generates resentment and ultimate dissatisfaction on all sides.

In the true help transaction, both the helper and the person receiving help get to *choose* what they want to give and receive. Free choice means satisfaction and success because each person senses his own participation. Neither is being forced to or inhibited from giving or receiving help.

Choosing to give and receive a particular kind of help establishes that the help transaction is between equals. Both the giver and receiver are doing exactly what they want to do.

Ultimately, people have equal power. You have some priceless knowledge and skills to apply to real problems. The people who have these problems, despite the problems, are equal to those of us who can help solve the problems.

And, finally, a patient's acknowledgment or thanks for help in solving a health care problem and our thanks to the patient for the opportunity to help bring a great deal of joy to the health care field. That, in fact, is what it's all about.

Your Health and the Patient's

IT CAN BE VERY CONVINCINGLY ADVANCED THAT YOUR MOST important duty as a person helping to solve other people's health problems is to be healthy yourself. By health here, though, I am referring to the attitude you have with yourself and the attitude that is communicated within the entire health care team. Those attitudes broadcast to the patient, to the family, to the rest of the primary care team, and to the public.

What constitutes a healthy attitude in the health care situation? First, stability, competence, and confidence born of knowing you have something to contribute to another person's plight. Second, knowing that you want to make those contributions that are wanted and really will help. Third, having absolutely full attention available for the patient. This latter, of course, is not possible if there are residual disagreements among your own team. Discomfort among your team broadcasts no matter how cleverly you may think the discomfort is disguised. Stress, uncomfortable boredom, antagonism, confusion, and frustration among team members is not only counterproductive, it actually is irresponsible of us in the sense that we are subjecting our patients to unnecessary suffering.

Staff Muck

Muck, the word I use to refer to that list of discomforts above, is common to every field of endeavor where people work together. Muck, by definition, is that feeling of discomfort that sometimes arises in our dealings with other people. Muck is an everyday phenomenon, even in some of our best teams. And muck is not in itself a problem. The potential problem lies in how we deal with it when it is there.

For an everyday phenomenon with the critical importance of muck, most of us have had little direct training or guidance, especially in our "formative" years, in how to deal with it. While our profession abounds in training in how to figure muck out, or analyze it, or categorize it, the fact remains that there is very little down to earth training in how to get rid of it constructively. Yet there it is, looking us straight in the face again and again, sometimes just a low-grade distraction but ranging up to a nearly consumptive frustration. And there we are, often left mainly to our own devices, to get ourselves out of our own discomfort. Because we are left to our own, often random, devices, we sometimes deal with muck effectively, that is, in ways that actually solve the problem, and we sometimes deal with muck ineffectively, that is, in ways that don't solve the problem, make the problem worse, or create bigger attendant problems. By and large, when we are being ineffective in dealing with muck we are using old habits: retreating from the muck or the situation we believe is causing the muck, avoiding the muck, or playing with the muck.

The Retreat

Jim and Gloria work together on the P.M. shift. Jim has had the persistent feeling lately that Gloria doesn't do her part, that he, Jim, ends up doing most of the work. He does it because he wants to do the best by the patients, but he is working with a slowly building resentment and an increasing sense of martyrdom. Jim has some muck. While he is being pretty clever about hiding his discomfort from his patients, still it spills over a little in the form of little side remarks, his indirectly communicated sense of being unjustly over-busy, his partial distraction, and, in general, a sense, which he inadvertently communicates, of being unjustly put upon. Rather than continuously remembering that he is working in the field of his active choice, Jim is feeling somewhat forced to make more contributions than he can or wants to, and he blames Gloria.

All of that communicates, albeit indirectly, to Jim's patients.

Jim tried to discuss the matter with Gloria, but the more he talked, the more indifferent she seemed to become, until finally, Jim slammed down his clipboard and bolted out of the room, in his mind justifiably frustrated past the point of tolerance by a fellow worker who was clearly wrong and not caring.

What Jim did was to retreat. Once in that room with Gloria he was reminded of his building frustrations. He left the room in the midst of muck in an attempt to get out of the muck, his own discomfort. A retreat, then, occurs when a person who is in the muck changes his physical situation or location *in an attempt to get out of the muck*. A retreat can be quite dramatic, as with Jim above, or it can be very subtle. In either case, the retreat will i) not solve the original problem, and ii) be followed by "new muck," no matter how radically we have changed our situation or location.

Retreats have this disadvantage to you: in the midst of a retreat we are muttering to ourselves, "never again." The things we swear to ourselves in these unfortunate moments are sometimes bizarre and always limiting. The extreme case is the person who, in the midst of the horrendous muck in his or her marriage, opts not to clear up the muck directly with whatever resolution will follow, but to leave the marriage in the midst of the muck as a solution to the muck. This person, then, is likely to mutter to himself in the midst of the retreat, "never again am I getting married." Whether he remembers this solemn oath or not, his ability to see people and relationships for what they are, one by one, is prejudiced indefinitely.

More importantly, the person retreating never sees how he is participating in the problem. He actually attributes the muck to the situation or to the other people, thereby sentencing himself to some version of his habitual mistakes in the future.

Any time a person is in the muck, in this example Jim and probably Gloria too, that person is participating in the problem in such a way as to help keep the problem and the muck there. That participation could be by omission, by not doing or saying something, or it could be commission, by actively doing or saying something that adds to the problem and the muck and thereby keeps it there. That participation must be there for the muck to remain.

Avoiding the Muck

Avoiding someone with whom or some situation with which you have muck not only doesn't solve the problem, it amounts to one of the biggest attention and energy drains you could devise for yourself. Imagine it. You have some muck or discomfort with your boss, and the muck seems to get worse every time you are around him or her. It just seems easier to avoid him, thereby avoiding that muck, right? Not really. Just think. What do you have to do to effectively avoid him? You have to not bump into him. But how do you know where not to go? Even more than not bumping into him, to *really* avoid him you have to not think about him. But how do you remember to not think about him without thinking about him? Ultimately, to effectively avoid someone you must keep track of him at all times. He has to be on your attention, somewhere in the back of your mind, at all times. In an extreme, you've got to keep track of this guy's lunch habits so that you can effectively avoid him during lunch hour. And the more you "must" avoid him, or the situation, or the emotion you have attached to him, or the thought, or the subject, or the elevators, or whatever, the more that person or thing is on your mind. And all that time your distraction and preoccupation is communicating to the very people to whom you want to communicate health, your patients.

Muck Pies

People sometimes get enamored with the process of doing away with muck, rather than focus on the result of having done away with it and getting back to actual work. That trap occurs when the goal is to be in "good communication," rather than *using* good communication to reach the goal of being in good teamwork on the job. People can make literally endless projects of "handling" things, with the resultant atmosphere of a nearly continuous encounter session, muck spilling out over everyone, including our unwitting patient, whose only sin was to get sick or injured.

      The assistant administrator, Ted, for example, is, in certain ways, a well-respected manager—so much so that people like to be around him, to learn, to get advice, to pick his brain, and so forth. But because of certain distractions outside of work Ted has recently fallen into the habit of only being accessible to his supervisors and department heads when they have a problem. Ted has built himself a trap. The more respected he is, the more people want to be around him. But the only way they can get to him is when they have a problem. What are the meetings going to be like? And Ted, for his part, is liking these meetings less and less because it always seems to be a hassle! In many subtle ways, then, Ted becomes less and less accessible to everyday communication, and in so doing, adds more bars to his own self-constructed cage.

Institutional Muck

Institutional green walls and tepid food do not communicate health and recovery. Blandness does not communicate life; it communicates boredom with life, the very phenomenon that probably contributed to the illness or injury to begin with. Processed and additive-afflicted foods served without attention to visual and olfactory attractiveness also do not communicate health and recovery. Rather, they communicate laziness and, frankly, unconcern or ignorance of a thickening body of evidence that nutrition and attitude have a great deal more to do with recovery than we as a profession have always thought and taught. Yet despite our collective habits, it remains true that hospitals, clinics, private offices, and homes with recovering patients have a responsibility to communicate health, not illness or those factors reinforcing illness. As much as possible, the physical surroundings of patients should be part of the solution, not add to the problem. We have all seen health care facilities that look more like interment institutions than physical spaces that help to communicate the steps toward recovery. The combination of drab surroundings, poor, tepid meals, and night noise (as if sleep or rest for the patient were less important than the staff keeping themselves entertained) can add up to a pretty convincing communication to patients, a sense that runs counter to healing and recovery.

The Personal Touch

Communicating health to patients includes relating to the patient as a person of equal power and ability to yours. The patient is not a victim of anything at all, at least in the sense of thinking of victims as "poor thems." The reality is that your patient is an equally able person who happens to have a problem. You have some priceless knowledge and skills to apply to that problem, and your place of work is hopefully ideally set up and equipped to help the patient to solve his problem.

Left Alone, Muck Grows

Having muck within the health care team or in parts of the team prevents complete trust within the team. Trust can be simply defined as complete confidence in another person's word or actions, the absence of worrisome attention. It is difficult to ask patients—people who are waiting, who sense danger and who feel fear already—to trust a group of strangers who do not completely trust each other. Therefore, the muck must go.

      The first step is to recognize that having muck in and of itself is not wrong as much as it is disadvantageous. Everyone I have ever met, several pretenders notwithstanding, gets himself or herself into the muck at times. To blame yourself for getting into the muck gets you no further than, for instance, Jim blaming Gloria, or his rank, or his background, or his sex, or his education, or his disadvantages in life for his muck. In Jim's case, since he thinks Gloria is to blame then Jim will have to wait for Gloria to change to get himself out of the muck! The more Jim is accurate that Gloria *is* contributing to the problem, the longer Jim's wait once he starts blaming Gloria. Blaming oneself leads to a different, but equally baffling, trap. Once you start blaming yourself, you feel bad. Then one day you recognize that you are blaming yourself and feeling bad about it. Now everyone knows he shouldn't blame himself, so he can only blame himself for blaming himself! A downward spiral. The actual fact is that getting in the muck is a very human thing to do—but so is getting out.

Recognizing one's own participation in mucky situations, objectively recognizing that participation, is quite different than blaming oneself or someone else or a situation for your plight. That recognition is, in fact, the gateway out of the muck. Then, and only then, can you see which on your list of complaints or dissatisfactions are attributable to yourself, and thus easily corrected, and which are attributable in part or in whole to the other people involved. To achieve this kind of objectivity, one must get the complaints and worries out of the mind, where they just rattle around and worry us more. Left in the mind, complaints and worries cause us to lose perspective. To start getting out of muck in a particular situation we therefore want to get the mucky contents out of our mind: for instance, down on paper. Look down the list to see how, by omission or by co-mission, you have been participating in the muck, or in allowing it to grow, or in allowing it to stay there. Look at that list of participation to see which of your habits here are easily corrected.

Hooks

Those ways we participate in making our own discomfort (i.e., "hooks") vary in as many ways as there are different people and different automatic habits in the world. Some hooks we have more or less in common with other people, and some are unique to each of us as an individual. One of the common hooks is to hesitate to express immediately what is really on our minds before it builds up. The justification for the hesitation or omission nearly always boils down to a fear of consequence, and the result of that hesitation is usually the actualization of some form of that, heretofore, only imagined consequence.

For example, Dr. Jones, an attending physician,

and Ms. Smith, a nurse, have developed together what has now become pretty nearly continuous failure to communicate clearly together. Ms. Smith started off doing pretty well in her communications with Dr. Jones, being direct and informative when appropriate. As was her comstom with previous physicians she had worked with, Ms. Smith would state her opinions *without undue force but also without undue fear and hesitation,* both when those opinions agreed with what seemed to be the plan and also when an opinion or piece of information might have caused a review and possible revision of the current treatment plans. In that way Ms. Smith was acting as a positive creative member of the health care team, making those contributions needed when a situation calls for maximum input before a direction is chosen or changed. At first Dr. Jones seemed to receive that input without undue reaction and he, therefore, was also acting as a positive and creative member of the team, actually listening to his team members and at times visibly using the information to the patients' advantage. But over the past several months Dr. Jones has appeared to Ms. Smith as distracted and irritated when information and opinions were offered. After several instances of this perceived behavior, Ms. Smith began to feel that her comments were not welcome and probably not even heard anyhow. Several other members of the team had the same impression and discussed that impression, not with Dr. Jones, but with each other when Dr. Jones was not around. On one occasion some months ago Dr. Jones actually blew up at Ms. Smith when she questioned a dosage prescribed on the ward by Dr. Jones. Ms. Smith's question had been posed tactfully, and, in her mind, his reaction had been rude and unjustified. Ms. Smith had no difficulty finding complete agreement among other team members for her feeling about Dr. Jones' reaction. Looking back now, Ms. Smith can see that from that point on she volunteered only the minimum information to Dr. Jones, often stifling her own heartfelt opinions about what might be best for a particular patient at a particular time. After all, who needs it?

Dr. Jones, for his part, feels utterly responsible for his patients' welfare, a responsibility he feels he shares with no one and, therefore, he has developed a sense of caring that has become almost burdensome to him. He has over the years become aloof, distracted, and easily irritated when questioned or when he imagines he is being challenged about a particular mode of care. His deepest fear, unidentified but nevertheless active within him, is getting discovered making an error in the care of his patients. He has, therefore, gradually become motivated in part by this fear of consequence, which of course will make much more probable the actualization of those heretofore imagined and feared consequences.

What are the hooks? They exist, as they nearly

always do, on both sides of what has now become a silent contest manifested by a communication gap that results in disharmony, albeit unspoken disharmony, and discomfort on this part of the health care team. Ms. Smith's holding back is perfectly justified, as hooks always are. In her mind, to talk frankly with Dr. Jones results in a flareup, which she doesn't want. Acting on or not acting because of that fear is the hook. Also, Ms. Smith has agreement from other staff, also justified, that Dr. Jones reacts at times irrationally. Obtaining and not acting because of that agreement is hook number two. Then, too, Dr. Jones appears distracted and disinterested and probably, in Ms. Smith's mind, doesn't want challenging or questioning information, and certainly wouldn't act on it anyhow. Hook number three. All of these hooks are perfectly justified, *and all result in Ms. Smith getting closer to the things she wants least:* a blowup on the ward, as mutual tensions mount toward the boiling point, and a compromise in care for the patient, as relevant information is withheld, communicated indirectly, or glossed over in an attempt to not rock the boat.

Dr. Jones' hook is his fear of making an error and being discovered. That fear is harmless in and of itself, but because of that fear, Dr. Jones has unknowingly developed an aura of unapproachability, relative inflexibility, and, at times, extreme irrascibility. This aura is pronounced enough to have gained Dr. Jones a silent reputation. Dr. Jones has forgotten how to receive information, and he therefore cuts off his best, besides the patient himself, sources of information, the people who actually take care of the patient. He, therefore, inadvertently advances one step further toward an actual manifestation of his worst fear, to not do the very best possible by his patients.

Both people, perfectly justified though they are, participate in erecting the communication and action obstacle. This part of the team, then, cannot act in complete harmony on the patients' behalf. Other members of the health care team get caught in the middle, listening to complaints from both sides.

Everyone has fears, hesitations, and reservations about certain types of communications to certain people in certain situations. The hesitations are not the problem. Acting or not acting because of those hesitations may, though, result in what we all want least: actual realization of our fears and a compromise to forming and maintaining great teams which result in the best patient care.

It's a nice profession: a vital first step in delivering the help we all want to deliver is to be healthy in attitude ourselves. It gives us an excuse, if you will, to have and maintain for ourselves that ingredient so valued in every aspect of our lives, a healthy attitude that leaves time and attention for someone else.

F   I   V   E

Tuning In

THE PATIENT'S POINT OF VIEW IS A LOT DIFFERENT FROM that of the person charged with his care. Being wheeled on a cart is a lot different from being the wheeler.

The explanation of the difference is simple. The experience of the difference is dramatic, sometimes traumatic.

The patient is the person actually experiencing the problem. He senses personal danger. He almost always is filled with dread because he feels his future is uncertain. He frequently is consumed by terror. He is immersed in the illness experience, and, for the moment, nothing else matters.

Caring for the patient, we are participating in his experience from the outside. The illness or injury is his, not ours. We are there by choice. We do not experience danger or dread or terror. We view the illness or emergency as a problem requiring a decisive solution, and we are immersed in providing that solution.

If we want to deliver the best care possible, we must find out all we can about the patient's situation. The expert in this is the patient himself, since he has had the direct experience. The starting point toward optimum care, then, is to assume the patient's point of view while simultaneously maintaining the objectivity of our own experience in handling the health care problem.

One valid approach toward assuming the patient's point of view is to ask yourself a question: *If I were the patient, what would I want from those delivering my care?*

I have asked this question of myself and of several thousand people involved in all aspects of health care. The answers are surprisingly similar. Most people seek safety. The patient senses danger, and he wants to be delivered from that danger safely. He wants assurance, the communication of competence and skill. He wants to know what is happening, the names and functions of the people attending him, information about what is going on at the moment and what he might expect in the immediate future. He wants compassion and understanding. He wants to feel that people are *interested* in him, not only as a problem but also as a person.

Consider the view from the gurney. The perspective is completely different from normal. This changed perspective is so difficult to imagine that I frequently ask people working in the Emergency Department or on the floor to actually *experience* it. I ask them to lie on a gurney, and I have them wheeled through the Emergency Department or from the floor to the O.R. It is an eerie sensation. Familiar rooms become frightening from that angle. After only a few minutes on the gurney, departmental professionals obtain a much more accurate perception of the patient's point of view.

I have seen this simple reminder of the patient's situation result in a hundred little miracles of compassion and understanding. After having been on the gurney themselves, attendants are more likely to keep actual patients informed what is happening. "We're going down the hall now, and then we'll turn to the right and get onto the elevator." Such information goes a long way toward relieving a patient's fear and apprehension.

Each coin has two sides. Our perception of the patient's experience will be enormously more accurate if we can adopt the patient's point of view, and as our ideas about his experience become more accurate, we will increase, tremendously, the accuracy and effectiveness of our treatment. On the other side of the coin, as the patient accepts our point of view of the potentials and limitations of health care, his perception of the situation and prospects will be more accurate. This increased accuracy will result in increased patient responsibility and better patient care as he makes himself more a part of the health care team.

In realizing your true intention to provide excellent care and to serve in your best capacity, the first step is to take the patient's point of view and, within the limitations of the situation, try to provide the things that the patient needs or wants. If you cannot accept his point of view, you cannot imagine his needs and wants. At the same time, you must maintain your point of view as a professional with the ability to maintain objectivity and utilize your own experience. This mixed viewpoint, carefully balanced, maximizes your responsibility and optimizes the final result.

The patient may be relatively disoriented to the present. He is, after all, in new surroundings, probably filled with unfamiliar instruments, people, and constantly changing dramas.

The unknown future frequently compounds a patient's disorientation. He does not know what can be done for his condition, how long it will take, whether there will be a disability, whether treatment will be painful, embarrassing, or expensive.

In dealing with the emergency or severely ill patient, we often are dealing with someone who is, to a greater or lesser degree, uncertain about what has happened, what is happening, and what might happen in the immediate future. We have termed this condition "relative disorientation," and it certainly must be considered in meeting the patient where he is, tuning in on his wavelength.

The overwhelming concern of the emergency or seriously ill patient is the stark reality that he is experiencing a crisis. He feels that he is in danger and that the danger holds the potential of serious personal loss. No matter whether the danger is real or imagined, major or minor, the patient senses *great* danger, and it is precisely that feeling, combined with the premonition of serious personal loss, which has brought him to us.

It is important to understand this because we cannot expect the patient to form a team with us in caring for his problem unless we appreciate his complaint *from his point of view*. It is a simple matter to tune in on the patient's wavelength when our conceptions of reality match, when the emergency is obvious, and when we and the patient agree without hesitation on the proper course of action. The inherent dangers are obvious when we are faced with severe lacerations, fractures, the life-threatening situations. One look is enough for the care team and the patient to identify the emergency problem. Then we can accept the challenge for the problem's solution. We can assure responsibility to minimize or eliminate the danger.

But we see many patients whose complaint is not so obvious. Many of us, in fact, are often bothered by what we consider nuisance cases—instances when there is obviously nothing wrong with a patient or instances when the objective complaint is so minor that we wonder why the patient ever came to us. We are frustrated and too often short-tempered in such cases because we cannot help solve a problem that is not real to us. It seems that we have nothing to offer.

In our irritation, we forget one important fact; the patient is there because he believes he is experiencing an emergency. He is *convinced* that he is in danger, that he faces the potential of a serious personal loss. Viewed objectively, the real or imagined danger may appear to us to be minimal or even silly, but this is only because we have failed to tune in on the patient's wavelength.

Failure to identify the patient's problem *as he sees it* almost always leads to a very unsatisfactory encounter. There is very little we can offer a patient whose problem has not been identified and therefore cannot be addressed directly. If the problem bothering the patient is not addressed, chances are he will persist in providing exaggerated or misleading information about his condition. This creates a stand-off. We become even more irritated by his irrational exaggerations, and he becomes more upset by our "lack of concern" and "off-hand attitude."

In these instances, I put myself in the patient's shoes and see his point of view regarding his problem and his ideas about the diagnosis or solution. In the beginning of the interview I tune in with him, at least temporarily. I align my point of view with his belief about his experience, however briefly.

The purpose here is to establish a common ground with the patient, to create at least some kind of initial identification of his problem. By acknowledging what is true for the patient in his emergency, we can provide him with an opportunity to accept our view of the situation and its solution. If he knows we are listening to him and understand, he will trust us and ultimately will permit us to deliver the real solution to the actual problem.

Example: A patient arrives in our department convinced that he has appendicitis. He has abdominal pain, and he feels that he might be in grave danger. He is afraid. Still, although he senses danger and fear, he may hesitate about verbalizing his problem. He may feel "silly" or unsafe about telling us that he has appendicitis. He may say only that he has a stomach ache. And we may diagnose his ailment, correctly, as the flu. But this question of appendicitis is the primary question he has come to have answered. If it is not answered, he will not be satisfied, and part of his problem will not be solved for him. As providers of care, we must find out why the patient feels endangered, what he thinks is wrong, what he thinks the worst could be, and what brought him to us in the first place. If we tune in with the patient, identify the problem *as he sees it,* and then substitute the imagined problem with the actual problem, we will have eliminated the danger experienced by the patient.

Another example: A patient arrives in our Emergency Department in an agitated state. His actions and attitude are very dramatic. This happens frequently and can be understood. An emergency is not a normal occurrence, and occurrences outside the normal often seem dramatic. There is the drama of the emergency situation itself, the screaming ambulance's rush to the Emergency Department, the reactions of the patient's friends or relatives, the unfamiliar movie-set atmosphere of the Emergency Department itself. It is not difficult to understand that a patient experiencing the drama of an emergency situation might act dramatically. And, in this instance again, it is best if we tune in on the patient's wavelength. He is the start of the drama. If we fail in our roles as supporting players, he might well feel that he has received less than adequate service. It should be easy for us to fall in with his dramatic view of the situation, since our plan of work as health care professionals very often actually are dramatic.

In attempting to meet the patient where he is, it is

important to realize that patients in nearly every emergency event are suffering greater or lesser degrees of unconsciousness. In an emergency, the spectrum of patient unconsciousness ranges from full unconsciousness or unawareness to mild reality shock.

Reality shock results from a sudden interruption of the normality of life. It frequently results in disorientation to the immediate past, to the pain, fear, and danger of the illness or injury.

Reality Shocks

EVERY PATIENT, AND PARTICULARLY THE EMERGENCY PA-tient, is experiencing to some degree a shock to reality. Most emergency patients, in my experience, resist the reorientation to reality which is necessary to minimize or eliminate the shock. Still, reality shock can be a major barrier to optimum care. It is a barrier which must be removed before we can hope to provide complete and successful patient care.

Reality is a person's experience of the way things are in his environment. It is colored by a person's *ideas* about reality, his *ideas* about the way things are or should be in his environment. A beautiful woman may have the *idea* that she is quite homely, and that is her reality. Man once had the *idea* that the world was flat, and that was his reality. Shock inevitably results when *ideas* about reality are smashed, when the actuality of reality or a person's perception of reality is suddenly changed.

Beginning with the illness or injury event itself, the patients we see daily experience a series of reality shocks. Each is snug and secure in the reality of his everyday environment when that reality is altered, suddenly and dramatically, by the illness or injury event: a finger is cut and blood flows; cars collide and bodies are damaged; a man suffers a sharp pain in the abdomen. Realities are shocked. Things suddenly are not as they were, not as they should be, not as they should have been. The patient experiences further reality shock in the emergency department, the ward or the office. He finds himself in new, strange surroundings, far from his conception of everyday reality. Further, his expectations of future realities are shocked; a future which seemed predictable before the event suddenly is doubtful and mysterious. Things will not be as they should have been, as they had been planned. There may be future pain, lengthy treatments, heavy costs.

Emergency and other patients, then, suffer reality

shocks in relation to the immediate past, the present, and the future. This results in past, present, and future disorientation.

Before we can deal effectively with the patient's condition, before we can obtain the patient's full cooperation and help him to respond responsibly after his initial treatment, we strive to reorient him to the realities of the past, present, and future.

Most patients, in my experience, initially resist such reorientation. They resist recalling the exact details of, for instance, the immediate event which resulted in the injury or illness.

Until recently, I considered this unimportant. Reorientation of the patient to reality seemed superfluous, for example, in the case of a patient with a laceration of the thumb who resisted recalling the exact circumstances of the knife slipping off the potato and cutting through the skin. In situations like a simple laceration or a minor illness, I thought it was enough to obtain the bare facts needed for diagnosis and treatment.

It is not enough. To the extent a patient is disoriented with his immediate past, to the extent that he still suffers reality shock in connection with the illness or injury event itself, he cannot give his full attention to his situation as a patient. This dispersal of attention diminishes the patient's ability to cooperate in his own treatment.

I have evolved a simple, conversational method of dealing with patient disorientation to the immediate past.

After appropriate introductions, I ask the patient a question: "Exactly what happened?" I simply receive and acknowledge any answers given, without making judgments or evaluations. When this question is answered, I ask: "What happened first?" Again, I accept the answer at face value and acknowledge it. I may repeat this question, or paraphrase it, until I know we actually are at the beginning of the event or illness. Especially in accident or critical situations, I have found it helpful to ask about the scene of the accident, where did it happen, who else was there, what was the patient doing or thinking at the time, what dangers were sensed. This questioning process sometimes must be repeated four or five times before the patient has fully remembered his experience of the event.

But when a patient finally is in touch with his *experience* of the event—as opposed to his *ideas* about the event—he is in a position to be more in control of his present situation. Then he can cooperate fully in his own care.

This questioning process sometimes makes patients temporarily uncomfortable. They may even protest. They think it will be difficult or even painful to recall the emergency event. But I have found that the patient's *idea* of the difficulty or pain that he expects to encounter is more frightening than the actual recall. I handle any protest by letting the patient know my purpose in asking the questions and asking for his cooperation. If the patient is unwilling to recall the event, I don't force it. This is quite rare.

The end result of this process is to give the patient an opportunity to communicate his thoughts, feelings, and reactions to his situation and to make them real in the real world. This memory rehabilitation removes disorientation to the immediate past.

Equally simple methods can be employed to eliminate patient disorientation to the present.

The present, for the patient, is his presence in the Emergency Department, the hospital floor, or your office. Most patients do not share your reality of, for instance, an emergency department. They are strangers surrounded by strangers, strange apparatus, and strange procedures. In addition, an emergency patient has the notion that he may have to witness some incredibly horrifying scene at any time during his stay there.

Patient orientation to the present should begin with the receptionist. She should indicate to the patient and relatives that they have indeed arrived at the right place, the place where their problem is "welcome." If the receptionist has a negative attitude or is harsh or abrupt in his or her initial dealings with the patient, he will feel that his problem is *not* welcome. He may then *dramatize* his problem beyond its actual proportions to make it big enough or important enough for the receptionist to notice. This you do not need.

The receptionist should be pleasantly efficient at all times. Most important, he or she must be informative and interested in the patient. On first contact with the patient, she actually can say: "This is the Emergency Department (or wherever). I am Mary Smith, and I will be asking you for information which we need to help take care of you." She also should point out the waiting room for relatives and non-urgent patients and indicate there will be a wait (if this is the case) and say *why* there will be a wait. She also should indicate the approximate length of the wait and say that at the end of that time someone will come out for them.

This is the beginning of patient orientation to the present, to place and time in the health care facility, to the people who are part of this new reality.

Every person who approaches the patient should tell him in a friendly manner just who they are, why they are there, and what is going to happen next. "Hi, I'm Mr. Jones, and I'm the nurse. I am going to take your temperature, pulse, and blood pressure to gain information for your care."

Any time the patient is moved from place to place, the reality of this move should be indicated to the patient.

The nurse meeting the patient in the waiting room should indicate the impending move to the examining room. It is not enough to say, simply, "Please come this way." The nurse should say: "We are going to another room for your first examination." If rooms do not exist, partitions of drawn curtains can be utilized to provide the patient with needed privacy.

The physician can orient the patient to the procedure of history, examination, and possible lab or x-ray studies. This elicits patient participation and helps eliminate the potential attitude that the patient is there to have something done *to* him. Proper procedure on the part of the physician also can eliminate assumptions that the patient is a victim, a body left at the mercy of a blood pressure cuff. Actually, the patient is a human being with a powerful will. He has the ability to take a measure of control and responsibility for his condition, its diagnosis, and possible remedy. And he is going to need that will of his intact as his primary means of recovery.

When the physician completes the history and physical examination, he may indicate that he is ordering lab tests or x-rays. I usually say that someone will be along to accompany the patient to the x-ray department, where an x-ray will be taken of the chest, and that I will talk again with the patient after I have read the films or got the report. If appropriate, I indicate a possible wait in the x-ray department. This builds orientation to immediate future events.

These all are simple and basic operating premises. These elements of orientation are so obvious as everyday operating procedures that one or more of them may be missing or inconsistently applied in your sphere of operations.

The importance of these procedures cannot be over-emphasized. Informative communication with the patient establishes and maintains orientation, continuity, and trust. Patients often hang on every word of Health Care personnel. If what you give them to hang onto is not stable, the patient will not feel stable, and you will be forced to deal with those extra feelings and emotions rather than simply getting down to patient care.

Orientation of the patient to the immediate future is as important as his orientation to the past and present.

The immediate future in a busy Health Care Center usually involves a wait. Wait for a nurse, wait for x-rays, wait for the physician, wait for lab results. When the waiting time is predictable, within limits, this can be communicated to the patient and relatives. When the wait is unpredictable, communication of this fact can help build patient orientation and relieve tension. He will *know* the waiting time is unpredictable, and will not fret as much about it.

Telling a patient how long he must wait for the next step or telling him that the waiting time is unpredictable simply removes some of the mystery from his immediate future. Removing mystery results in increased patient presence, participation, and responsibility. This results in better health care when the patient leaves us and resumes full responsibility for his own problem.

A brief talk with the patient as he is leaving the care of your facility can further his orientation to the immediate future. I have found it useful to discuss the beginning, middle, and end of the health care transaction during such summaries, and say something like: "Well, (1) you came here with such-and-such a problem, and (2) we did such-and-such while you were here and reached these conclusions and obtained these results, and (3) now you've finished here and will be seeing Dr. Smith in follow-up. Do you have any questions?"

This emphasizes what the problem was, how we assumed temporary responsibility for the patient's problem, what is the problem's present status, and how the patient can get more help and resume full responsibility for his problem.

All of these techniques in handling patient disorientation to reality may seem very time-consuming. Actually, I have found these techniques are substantial *time savers*. As they become a part of normal procedure, these techniques take only seconds to apply. The service that you render a patient in following these techniques is immeasurable.

Health Care Beliefs

BOTH THE PATIENT AND THE HEALTH CARE PERSONNEL temporarily responsible for his care arrive at the medical transaction steeped in a formidable array of beliefs.

Because these beliefs can produce unwanted problems and conflicts on both sides of the transaction, it is worthwhile to briefly consider the nature of belief.

A belief is an acceptance of something as true without direct experience or knowledge. If we think of all reality, all proven facts as being contained in a circle, belief is what we feel to be true outside that circle. Belief, therefore, is sustained by faith and assumption, rather than perception.

The first step in forming a belief comes in an attempt to explain a phenomenon about which we have insufficient or false information. If a phenomenon does not make complete sense, we tend to want it to make sense anyway. We are willing to take things for granted, to suppose, to fill in what is missing. We make *assumptions.*

An example: A person comes in from the rain, and he is sneezing. This much is information. It is human nature to want to explain the information to reduce the mystery of what causes what. So we fill in the blanks between pieces of objective information; we assume that he caught a cold by being out in the rain. Others present have heard of this association and *agree* with the assumption. A conclusion is reached, a decision made, a belief formed or reinforced. The root of the word "decision" means to "cut, cut off" and implies cutting off doubt and wavering or forcing a conclusion. Assumption, agreement, decisions, and conclusions are the structure of belief.

Each new event occurring in relation to a certain belief adds structure to that belief in the form of additional assumptions, agreements, and decisions made by ourselves and others. After a while, this belief becomes a fixed part of the way we relate to the world. It may become so fixed that we accept it as a stable reality, a reality that we resist losing.

As we mature, we look for what works to stabilize our experience of life and make it more predictable. We accumulate beliefs with associated assumptions, agreements, and decisions. We gather many beliefs associated with our bodies and personal welfare, since it is through our physical senses that we experience much of life. We forget we have many of these beliefs, yet they operate daily and with the same firmness as if we consciously remembered each one. In terms of everyday life, our understanding of our reactions and behaviour is decreased. This is because we are operating from forgotten decisions which may or may not be appropriate to situations apparently similar to those which first prompted the belief.

We may fear that loss of belief would lead to randomness and confusion in an area we had thought completed, harmonized, or stabilized. Rather than experience this uncertainty, we often prefer to have a predictable answer, even if it means limiting our viewpoints and experience.

Patients enter health care facilities with beliefs about what has happened to them, what is happening, and what will happen. These beliefs come from past experiences, assumptions, agreements, and decisions. They may or may not apply to the patient's present situation, but to the extent these beliefs have become firm and fixed, they will be the patient's operational base.

Firmly based beliefs diminish experience. The patient who sticks fixedly to a remembered or unremembered belief will, to that extent, be unable to experience what actually is happening in *this* circumstance, at this time, in this place.

On the other side of the transaction, we, in health care, are not without our beliefs about patients. There often is a temptation to make snap judgments or jump to conclusions based on incomplete observations which agree with seemingly similar situations in the past. We settle any remaining doubt by jumping to a conclusion regarding the patient. This sequence is common and insidious, and when a medical condition is missed or inaccurately diagnosed, this insidious sequence frequently is at the bottom. The dangers are obvious.

At the same time, our beliefs about social strata, race, sex, age, ability to pay, past medical history, emotional overlay, and a hundred other ingrained beliefs can blind us to noticing fully what actually is happening at this time, in this place, with this individual.

In health care we must be as objective and observant as possible, careful that we are guided by the facts as we see them rather than by our personal beliefs.

Victims:
Who Are They?

MOST OF US ARE INVOLVED IN HEALTH CARE, ESSENTIALLY, to help. Basic to all that we do, despite the humdrum and sometimes frustrating everyday routine, is the hope of experiencing the immense satisfaction of contributing to the well-being of others. At the end of the day, most of us like to feel we have contributed something to someone, somewhere.

The truth of the matter is that in realizing the satisfaction of contributing to others, we are satisfying ourselves. It is sometimes embarrassing to admit this, but the contribution to our own self-satisfaction is what keeps health care going.

I define help as contributing to our own or another person's well-being.

Some approaches to patient care are actively not helpful to either the patient or the person temporarily in charge of his care. It usually helps neither the patient nor ourselves, for example, when we assume a "bleeding heart" attitude. There is nothing essentially wrong with this attitude, except that it simply doesn't work to produce satisfaction on either side of the health care transaction.

Some of the philosophy of modern health care, and particularly crisis or emergency health care, evolves from the point of view of saving victims. Use of the word victim is common. The victim concept implies that fate caused the event to occur and that it is our responsibility to rescue the victim from his fate. Whether or not this is true, it tends to rob the patient of respect and of whatever responsibility he may be able to assume for the cause of his problem and for the effect it is having on him and will continue to have on him as his health improves. For a patient to be or become comfortable with the ultimate responsibility for the outcome of a condition of his own body does not imply that the patient is to blame for the existence of the condition.

If we insist on approaching the patient with the attitude that we are saving a victim, we must assume that the patient

35

has little or no responsibility for the outcome. This attitude makes us look like knights on white chargers, but it also causes us to push care toward the patient rather than work with him as a team to produce the results desired by both.

Actually, the patient and the persons delivering his care are equals, involved in solving the same problem from their respective points of view. Adoption of this point of view optimizes the patient-care result.

This approach to the patient as a person experiencing a problem in his health, rather than as a victim of fate who needs our rescuing efforts is simple and workable, yet as a consistent approach, it is unusual.

Far from robbing us of the opportunity to help, this point of view greatly enhances our ability to produce real help. Real help enhances the well-being of an equal. Real help is an action, inaction, or transaction which maintains or alters existence for another person in a desirable manner.

The key word here is *desirable*. Desirable for whom? For us? For the patient? For both?

If we are really helping the patient, we are contributing to the well-being of both the patient and ourselves. So we must decide what is desirable in the situation for both the patient and for ourselves.

Most of us agree that certain priorities, such as preserving life, are mutually desirable. Apart from such obvious benefits, we can discover what is desired by the patient only by asking and listening to the patient's point of view about what he wants. No matter what priorities and assumptions we might be tempted to make, no matter the dictates of our own knowledge and experience, only the patient knows what he considers desirable to maintain or alter his own existence. In my experience, nothing is more frustrating than seeking one kind of help and finding the helper trying to force an entirely different kind of help. It often is a kind of help neither desired nor needed.

When we, as the deliverers of health care, assume that we always know, ahead of time, what is best for the patient, we are robbing the patient of the opportunity to be responsible for as much of his health as he really can. This results in two undesirable effects: (1) the patient understands that the way to manage this situation is to "leave the driving to the doctor;" (2) he then may withdraw or diminish his active participation in the health care transaction and withhold communications which, if delivered, could add to the information available about the patient's condition. This diminishes the patient's responsibility and increases the potential for the patient blaming medicine for his condition or you for the outcome. And blame often results in patient passiveness, complaints, less improvements in health, and lawsuits.

Disease and Its Witnesses

ALL OF US IN HEALTH CARE NEARLY EVERY DAY ARE RE-quired to deal with patients who seem to us to be over-dramatizing their situation. The maudlin drunk, the whining pain presentation, the child with the temper tantrum, the patient threatening violence, and those patients dramatizing their sense of social or domestic victimization, to name a few.

This kind of presentation represents a potential danger to everyone involved: to the people trying to help; to the patient who may be obscuring a potentially consequential physical problem with his antics; and to the patient's family. The dangers to the patient and the family have been covered elsewhere in this book, and it is, therefore, the danger to us to which I address myself here.

The genesis of dramatic disease may actually be rather simpler than commonly thought. Dramatic disease is one of the end points, or final results, for a person who has forgotten what he really wants in life. The process of forgetting what one wants begins early in life with a communication problem, develops into a problem with fear, and ultimately becomes a problem of common sense mental capacity.

Hidden Standards

Let us say, for example, that Jim, who will become our patient a few years hence, is busily developing a habit that will result in a dramatic disease. Jim has started and is now continuing to develop the habit of not directly asking those around him for what he wants. He is developing the fear of rejection, a fear rampant in our society and yet totally not grounded in reality.

In his teenage years, Jim was attracted to Betty. Since a lot of the other kids were starting to date it occurred to Jim to ask Betty to the dance. But every time Jim thought about asking

Betty out, a thousand reasons occurred to him about why she would not be interested. So far in the story Jim is having an experience common to virtually all of us, be he man or woman. Over and over again every day of our lives, we have a choice between two sets of ideas, both sets of our own making: acting on an inclination to participate in a particular instance or not acting in that instance based on our fears or hesitations about the imagined consequences of that participation. Although he didn't consciously know it at the time, Jim was acting on the fears. So he never asked Betty out to the dances, but rather would lurk around the fringes of the dance hoping to bump into Betty but never actually causing that to happen. Jim was, therefore, perpetuating his habit, probably started much earlier in life, of choosing the fear and further assigning control over to thinking or worrying rather than acting purposefully.

Jim continued to allow this habit to dictate his success or failure in several arenas in his life for many years, not only with women that he felt attracted to, but whom he thought were better than he or would otherwise reject him, but also in certain career situations where he felt judged. In these instances, he would keep his brightest, most innovative, and possibly controversial ideas to himself, fearing one thing or another that added up to fears of losing friends, face, status, or even the job itself. As this habit got more ingrained and automatic, the fears became more and more real. In a kind of mechanism to avoid the fears attendant to identifying what he wanted, Jim became less and less conscious over the years of what he really did want in his heart of hearts, and how he really felt about things.

Jim's silence in these areas eventually led to his sense that "no one is listening." Soon, of course, no one *was* listening, for as Jim became more bored with himself and his own worries, he became more and more boring to be with. He began losing his audience, a direct result of his acting on the fears of losing that audience.

As one observes the life and activity around him, it becomes clear that everyday interactive life consists of a balance between participating, or being "on the stage," and watching others participate, or "being in the audience," as someone else talks with us, shows off for us, cooks for us, advances his or her ideas to us, or otherwise creates something for us to appreciate. Human beings need that balance of input and outflow for happiness, for a sense of control and, I submit, for physical health.

The Cough Drop

As Jim's case of the jitters advanced, it took more and more work for him to generate an audience. As he communicated less and less directly, he dramatized more and more loudly, in an unknowing attempt to recapture his audience. If he were with a group of people and he suddenly developed a cough, for instance, he would dramatize the cough rather than ask for a cough drop, again fearing that no one would have one, or that no one would give it to him even if they did have one, or that if people were really paying attention to him, they would *see* him coughing, know that he needed a cough drop, and offer one. But more and more, Jim felt that no one was catching on to his automatically dramatized but never actually directly communicated needs. So Jim dramatized more loudly, in this simple analogy to cough more, by now maybe even bringing up some stuff, hoping that someone would catch on and actually feeling that he *was* expressing his needs but that no one cared. And so it went with Jim, until dramatic illness became one of the last resorts in his unknowing attempts to recapture an audience that would appreciate what he needed. Of course by this time, Jim's communication habits had resulted in his own nearly total confusion about what it was that he actually did want. Jim was, in fact, developing into one of those personalities trying to figure out "who I am."

There is No Risk in Rejection

Actually, there is a risk in being direct about what you want in life, but that risk is not in rejection, it is in acceptance. Take Jim's cough drop for example. Let us suppose that he actually did ask for the cough drop and that he did not get it. Perhaps someone had one, maybe even showed it to Jim, and still wouldn't give it to him. So he did get rejected, in the way we usually think about rejection. But something else happened, too. At first Jim was coughing and didn't have a cough drop. Then he asked for it, and he didn't get it. Then he was still coughing and still did not have a cough drop. What had changed? One thing and only one thing had changed. Jim now knew for sure that if he really wanted a cough drop, he wasn't getting it in that group of people. He discovered "gravity." Now, far from being buried under the problem, Jim would be in an excellent position. For the first time in the entire interaction Jim would now be in a position to think creatively about his problem with this cough. Previous to this moment, Jim's only solution to his cough was that someone would miraculously catch on that he needed a cough drop and save him. After all, anyone really paying attention should see that he needed one (Jim's hidden standard). Except that didn't work. In not asking, Jim remained in his own self-constructed trap, having trapped himself into hoping that someone would catch on and in the meantime escalating the drama to ever more "obvious" proportions, hoping somewhere inside of himself at every increased level of drama, that this would be the step that would lead to his being saved. But as soon as Jim has asked directly, making sure people understood what he wanted, Jim has sprung his own trap. If he gets "rejected," he now knows that if he really wants to solve his coughing problem, he is going to have to think of something else besides getting a cough drop from someone in that room. *And that is the key to the creative thinking process in any endeavor.* That process starts only now, when we spring the trap of hoping without acting directly and purposefully. Now, if he wants to solve the problem rather than have the cough, he must think of alternative solutions to the coughing problem. Maybe a drink of water, some tea with honey, or something else would help this cough, thinks Jim, as he switches gears from self-made victim to a human being acting on his own behalf and, therefore, in a position to help others along the way.

Then What is the Risk?

I have advanced the idea that there is no risk in rejection. There certainly is *some* perceived risk in these situations, a perception undeniable given the way we all sometimes feel when we are confronted with asking for what we want. But that perceived risk does not have its ground in not getting what we want; it has its ground in our getting what we want. For then, when we are getting enough cough drops—enough love, appreciation, security, or whatever—then we must give something up: the right to complain, even to ourselves. That part of us, a large part in some, smaller in others of us, the part that feels the victim, that part gets fed only on self-made complaints, actionless hope that starts with a hidden standard. It is, therefore, giving up the *habit* of complaining to one's self and in advanced cases to others, the *habit* of acting out fear that constitutes the perceived risk. Those habits are so long-standing in most of us that they have become a modus operandus as second nature to us as brushing our teeth. Depending on how entrenched that habit has become, some people will exchange nearly anything to retain the right to complain justifiably, the right to commandeer an audience with the most justified imaginable complaint, that of physical illness, and particularly those special conditions I have termed dramatic illness.

The Danger to the Health Care Worker

The dangers to those who want to help are twofold: i) that having noticed the overly dramatic presentation, we assume the condition is limited to drama. That, of course, would lead to our missing some potentially serious conditions, as we take all claims and complaints from the patient as just so much attempt to gain attention. That happens when we forget that every patient has an emergency, even though he may be grossly misrepresenting himself. And, ii) the danger that we, ourselves, automatically bent on curing everyone, get frustrated in trying to help someone who has already decided— decided at one unremembered time quite consciously—that he would rather have the drama than have his health. The danger to the health care worker is not that we extend the best help available, which we are quite properly enjoined to do in every case, but that we get frustrated when this extension of help is rejected outright or seems to fall on barren ground. That frustration leads to boredom and a sense of burnout concerning the contributions we are trying to make. A certain cynicism is close behind.

It is our responsibility to offer and extend help and understanding fully, even walking the last mile. Further, it is our responsibility to recognize that not everyone will accept our offer, depending on what they really, in their heart of hearts, want. And further, it is our responsibility to understand these cases and not get frustrated ourselves. For in that frustration it is common and ex-tremely damaging to start drawing conclusions about people in general, or all men, or all women, or all "welfare"recipients, or all people in any category. At that point, our patients are not getting the individual and generous attention they each need and deserve as people and we, in the health care field, are "inexplicably" experi-encing a job that has somehow become not fun anymore.

Life Crisis and Patient Motivation

THROUGH THE YEARS SCORES OF VOLUMES AND PAPERS have been written on the subject of motivation. Much of that writing has served to complicate the subject so that motivation has become so shrouded in mysteries and unknowns that virtually everyone in the field admits to confusion. Yet for us in health care, it is essential to understand motivation, since without the factors of direction, determination, and persistent will, most of the very sick people we are trying to help are not going to do well. For the health care provider to achieve a thorough operational understanding of motivation, he or she need only take a simple direct view of motivation and apply that view to himself and what motivates him. When you really do understand what motivates you, you have something that will apply in basic terms to nearly everybody.

The Purposes of Human Energy

People make their own energy, moment to moment. While no one seems quite sure of how this is done, it does appear clear that our energy does not come from our bodies alone or from what we eat for breakfast or from our backgrounds or what our mothers told us about life. It also appears clear that we make activity energy in order to achieve certain purposes. If one morning you wake up and just can't seem to rustle yourself out of the sheets, chances are you have nothing to look forward to that day. Or you have something to look forward to that you wish weren't there! Throughout our day we oscillate between high activity energy states and low, depending on our individual ability to generate positive anticipation of our future, immediate or long term. So our lazy morning person will manage to get himself out of bed if he has generated a desirable future, even if that desired future is limited for then to the prospect of hot coffee, bacon and eggs.

In general, this is a good working hypothesis: *people make active energy in order to achieve desired futures, long term or short.* Therefore, to achieve and maintain a high state of motivation one needs at least the ingredients of i) vision, or the ability to postulate and ii) consciousness of his or her purposes. Will and determination then follow naturally.

Vision: The Desired Future

What constitutes a desired future for people? Again, turning to yourself as an expert reference, most readers will find that their desired futures will include the factors of i) challenge, or not knowing how things will come out, ii) the satisfaction that comes from *completing* cycles of activity, iii) the recognition that in achieving the anticipated goal someone else or others will be better off (i.e., will be contributed to) and iv) that the contribution will be received and recognized and some form of thanks extended.

Motivating Another Person

It is not possible to motivate another person. Attempts to do so will lead to your own frustration and eventual de-motivation, as it is not a desirable future for most to tackle something that can absolutely never progress. You can, however, make the enormous contribution of creating the atmosphere and opportunity for another person to motivate himself, and therein lies one of the most critical parts of your job as a provider in any capacity of health care. To provide that opportunity is as simple as it is critical, once one understands and applies the simple principles of motivation derived from studying yourself.

The Patient and His Purposes

People often forget that they have made purposes in life. A busy executive, for instance, caught up in the business and stress of a responsible position, may forget for years running that one of the purposes of his working so hard is to show love and support for his or her children. It is quite understandable, then, that at age 55 the executive's primary regret is that he did not spend as much time as he wishes with his children when they were young. That lapse did not occur because he doesn't like his children; it occurred because *he forgot one of his purposes.* Nevertheless, for years he has limited himself in his satisfaction in life by losing sight of the forest, his children, by being enmeshed in the trees of hurry, business, pressure, impatience, and his fears of insecurity. If he wakes up in time, he may be able to create the opportunity for achieving the satisfaction he missed with his young children by genuinely enjoying his grandchildren.

People who are sick are even more vulnerable to forgetting their purposes. Anyone who considers himself as really sick or injured may very quickly forget his goals, forget the contributions he or she is attempting to make and actually be revolted by, not attracted to, the everyday challenges of life. In short, many patients find themselves oriented toward death, or hopelessness, rather than life, or positive motivation.

Part of our job, then, is to remind patients, *always through questions* rather than statements or uninvited advice, to remember their purposes in life, to remember their "audience," those the patient wishes to contribute to, to remember the satisfaction in completing their current cycles, and to consider converting their illness from a tragedy to a personal challenge. When the patient remembers these things, chances are good that he or she will develop or redouble their will and their determination, ingredients they will need in their struggle to live or to die with grace and satisfaction.

Should I Tell Him?

It is often difficult for physicians to decide whether or how to convey to a patient a diagnosis that has a statistically devastating prognosis. Most physicians in my acquaintance have reached a moderately uncomfortable equilibrium in the position that they will level with patients in most circumstances, at least to the extent necessary to help the patient know that he must "settle his affairs." I believe myself that, under most circumstances, this approach has the most merit as long as the physician is careful to exclude absolutely his own sense of hopelessness about the prognosis. Regardless of the statistical prognosis in a given condition, we are all aware of the thousands of "miracles," or spontaneous remissions, that occur in virtually all conditions. These miracles, I submit, are the products of determined, willful, purposeful patients who never accepted the hopelessness of their statistical prognosis.

Those crestfallen and unctuously sympathetic facial expressions don't work either. There is nothing more disheartening to a newly diagnosed cancer patient, for instance, than to be greeted by the new nurse, physician, or clerk's suddenly sunken expression on learning that the new patient's diagnosis is cancer. That health care provider might as well be saying to the patient, "Oh, no, you're really in for it now," and the patient, if he (foolishly) trusts that health care provider's subtly transmitted opinion might as well hang it up right now.

We must be realistic in our communications to very sick people, but we must at the same time spare our patients our own subjective sense of dread, disaster, or hopelessness. Inform the patient, yes, and then help the patient orient himself toward challenge, toward completion, and toward contribution. Live or die, that patient then has the opportunity to remember something about why he or she came to life in the first place. And in that opportunity lies the contribution that disease has for the human race.

Using Your Head: Perception vs. Evaluation

THE ABILITY TO MAKE THE DISTINCTION BETWEEN PERCEP-
tion and evaluation on an everyday working basis is the single most
important skill in providing health care.

Perception is the process of collecting informa-
tion from the environment, done largely through the body. Perception is a first *unevaluated* impression.

Evaluation is the process of refining perceptions
into "knowledge." An evaluation is our idea about a particular
perception after we have applied to the original perception our personal judgment based on past experience.

We receive perceptions through our senses. We
see, hear, touch, smell, and taste. Some would allow for a sixth, in-
tuitive, or "natural knowing" sense, which I think is admissible for
the individual observer who is quite accomplished in separating
spontaneously his or her perceptions from the always-ready-to-
interfere evaluation apparatus of the human mind. That ability to
separate spontaneously can be re-learned by most people, once he
or she becomes disciplined and practiced in methodically
separating perception from evaluation. A strong first step is to
achieve an operational understanding of the mind's mechanism of
evaluation with an eye to applying that understanding to one's
everyday observations and conclusions. The second step is
disciplined practice, which leads in part to the rehabilitation of one
of your most valuable perception tools: your natural intuition to
know which of your conclusions "don't fit."

Once received through the senses, perceptions
are instantaneously fed into a memory vault through a computer-
like "first categorization" mechanism. This is how that first
categorization mechanism works: we see something and the
memory vault is flashed a perception of a certain shape. More
perceptions follow, almost instantaneously; the shape has a certain
size and volume. It has a distinctive texture. The memory vault, even

while receiving further perceptions, begins the process of evaluation. The first perception was one of shape. The memory sorts out objects of similar shape and presents a tentative identification of the perception. *The more perceptions observed and received by the mind before conclusions are drawn, the more positive will be the resulting associations, identifications, and conclusions.*

Again, the sorting process in most cases is instantaneous, and it depends upon a mental collection of past experiences with which this new perception can be compared. Amassing this collection and organization of data is one of the main purposes for the training we have received and are receiving. The amassed data and its organization explain the old saw "experience is the best teacher," for this part of the mind remembers experience much more distinctly than it remembers information collected didactically.

As an example, suppose the first impression or perception is something in the shape of a chair. The mind flips through its collection of past experiences and advises that the object is a chair. It is not a sofa, settee, davenport, or chaise lounge; it is a chair. *More perceptions make the identification more positive.* The back and seat of the chair consist of a single piece of bent plywood. The chair has three aluminum, rubber-tipped legs. The chair's plywood back is shaped somewhat like a lyre. The mind flashes these identifications and evaluations of perceptions after sorting through similar perceptions of the vast memory vault. The memory itself provides the final evaluation. This chair was seen in the design collection of the Museum of Modern Art in New York. It is a Charles Eames chair.

Exactly the same process operates in patient care. Perceptions coming mainly from objective historical information and the physical examination are sorted and compared with previous experience and knowledge. The more perceptions received by the mind, the more positive the final identification.

To the extent that we collect perceptions completely, we present the mind with maximum available objective information. By collecting complete perceptions and information, we minimize the danger of jumping to conclusions and committing ourselves to a treatment plan that is less than optimum. This premature conclusion process occurs when we automatically insert *opinions or assumptions or hopes or judgments* to part of our perceptions before the whole can be considered by the full categorization capacity housed in the mind. Here, in this premature conclusion process, a part of the mind automatically intrudes on the organization process, usually resulting in an inaccurate conclusion and a relatively "closed mind" on that subject at that time. The part of the mind I allude to here is the part which seems to insist, quite automatically, on drawing conclusions whether or not sufficient objective data are available (See Chapter on *Beliefs*).

The process of evaluating perceptions is further complicated by the fact that not all the data stored in the mind is available for use in the evaluation process. The mind's stored data, for our purposes here, can be discussed in three categories:

(1) Known and remembered data that is useable on a day-to-day basis.

(2) Data that is not remembered and, therefore, unknown. It is not accessible for use.

(3) Data which is known and remembered, but which carries such an emotional charge that it cannot be used to compare perceptions. This category is the root of *prejudice* in our health care judgments. Use of this data results in *automatic* snap judgments that are made without utilizing anywhere near the perceptions available in each individual case.

Comparisons in this last category raise a red flag when the incoming perceptions are identified. The mind tells us that the situation indicated by the perception is similar to one that was considered dangerous or threatening in our past experience. The mind presents this memory of danger so that we are alerted to check whether a similar danger is inherent in the present situation. The safest, most common assumption would be that the past danger might be present in the new situation, particularly when our individual mind is in stress. As a result, we often look at new situations through a kind of screen thrown up by past experiences and our reaction to them. This screen cuts off or changes perceptions which we otherwise would make more objectively.

All of us in health care have an obligation to arm ourselves with as much useable knowledge as possible. This means we must strive to expand the area of the first category above, where comparisons with experience are known and remembered and available for day-to-day use. Conversely, we must work to release data stored in the second and third categories; things that we once knew but have forgotten and comparisons which perhaps needlessly blind us to the truth by "warning" us of dangers that objectively do not exist in the present.

Taking the Mystery Out of the Vague Complaint

EVERY PATIENT WHO COMES TO US SAYING THAT HE IS EX-
periencing a crisis is indeed experiencing a crisis.

The patient's complaint may appear minor. He
may not appear ill or injured at all. He may be unwilling or unable to
identify the complaint. Still, he is experiencing a crisis whether he
has accurately identified or named that crisis or not. He would not
be looking for help if he did not sense potential danger to his own
well-being.

All of us involved in health care are acquainted
with this type of situation. Personally, I find it a real inconvenience
to interrupt a busy agenda or maybe even a between-events rest to
handle something that appears to be ridiculously minor. Most people in health care, I think, would agree. Handling minor or vague
complaints is one of the more frustrating aspects of our work. We
frequently become upset with the situation, with the patient, or with
ourselves.

There is nothing wrong with getting upset. In fact,
it can be thoroughly appropriate and even enjoyable at times. Getting upset, however, does not solve the problem.

A more workable approach is to analyze the problem. First, how is the situation a problem for me?

For example: Beyond the inconvenience and the
gut feeling that this is not really an emergency, I am disturbed by
such situations because I don't know what kind of help I am being
asked to supply. The patient is vague about his complaint. He is unwilling or unable to communicate his fears. I do not know whether I
can or will want to deliver the kind of help that may ultimately
emerge as wanted. I have no idea what I am trying to handle, let
alone whether I can or want to handle it. I don't know what to do to
help, so frequently, and sometimes gruffly, I want to get rid of the
situation.

The analysis of the problem from the viewpoint of

the person delivering health care leads to a solution. We can adopt the viewpoint of the patient and help him identify and communicate his complaint.

I have learned to approach the patient as if he is actively wondering or worrying about something. He always has at least one major question which, for him, is unanswered. That is why he has come for help. The answer to that question will remove the mystery surrounding the danger sensed by the patient in experiencing his problem. As professional health care personnel, we may agree to disagree that the danger is real. But we must remember: *The danger is real to the patient.* He is experiencing a crisis and that is why he has found us. He wants help.

We can supply the kind of help that is needed by assisting the patient in identifying the complaint and fear. Simple identification of the danger and the questions related to it strips away the mystery from the vague complaint, and the situation improves for the patient.

I have found it most effective to deal with this type of situation by asking direct questions. "What is your greatest concern here? What do you think is the worst possibility?" The exact wording of the questions is unimportant compared to the intention of asking questions that will help the patient remove the mystery from his experience.

Identifying the kind of help the patient needs or wants and determining whether we can supply that kind of help clears up many of the otherwise frustrating transactions in health care.

An example: A patient came to the Emergency Department because he had been hit in the eye with a tennis ball. The department staff had just finished handling two major emergencies, and everyone had adjusted their "emergency thermostats" to a high level, ready to handle highly challenging problems. This eye complaint seemed very insignificant to everyone. Everyone, that is, except the patient. He was acutely aware of the danger of losing his eyesight, a danger that was *real to him* and, therefore, real in a most relevant sense.

The technician who saw the patient first, attempting to reassure the patient, made light of the condition. This attitude made sense to the technician who had just been involved in two very serious emergencies. Levity, however, made no sense to the patient. This patient's problem was the most serious emergency in the universe for him. The patient got upset. In talking with him later, I found that the technician's attitude, although it was an attempt to help, had made the patient feel *he* was not being taken seriously. The patient's point of view, his fear of losing his eyesight, may have been uninformed. Yet it was real to him, and the technician's attitude did not match the seriousness of the patient's reality.

A lightly reassuring attitude was not the kind of help desired by this patient. What works in this type of situation is *matching* the patient's attitude of seriousness. This does not mean *agreeing* with him that the condition is serious. It means, in this case, receiving his point of view about the condition without placing evaluation on it for him (making it more or less serious, for instance). It means letting him have his point of view and letting him know you understand the seriousness he assigns to it. At that point, when the patient sees that his seriousness is matched, he is able to identify, consciously, the danger he feels; as in the example above, he might lose his eyesight.

We then conducted a thorough examination to confirm or eliminate all the potential dangers, including the one he felt was real. Then I communicated the findings, conclusions, and proposed treatment, including what he could expect in the immediate future. He then told me that what had been serious to him was the *potential* of danger. Once the danger was confirmed or eliminated, he knew, within limits, what to expect and how to take responsibility for it. He could then form a team with me and with the follow-up ophthalmologist to start to clear the eye condition.

The same concern for the patient's viewpoint is important in handling the anxiety or panic reaction.

I have developed a practical nuts and bolts approach toward the patient experiencing an acute anxiety reaction. This approach is not a therapy or necessarily a permanent solution. It does work predictably, however, to clear away the anxiety so that any physical problem accompanying the reaction can be more completely identified and treated.

The patient experiencing panic is unable to identify, consciously, the potential dangers which are real to him, but which he senses only vaguely. By simply identifying these dangers consciously, the patient can begin to settle down. Then we can see more clearly what kind of help is being asked of us and what parts of this help we can and cannot supply.

I asked: "What is the worst possible thing that this condition could mean for you?"

The purpose of this type of question is to give the patient the opportunity to identify and express the dangers he feels might underlie his condition. It is not an attempt to psychoanalyze the patient. My interest is to identify the immediate problem so I can do my job of ruling out organic disease.

He replied: "I might die; I might go balmy; I might have an auto accident; I can't take care of my store." I received and verbally acknowledged these answers without evaluation, for my evaluations could only interfere with the patient's ability to identify. Since I did not see any improvement in the patient, I repeated the question. He replied: "I might be humiliated." This answer was accompanied by a full and lasting smile on his face. I received this answer and then repeated back to him all the answers he had given me, in his words, as a means of assuring him that I had indeed received his answers.

I then asked him: "How are you doing right now?" He said he was feeling "better."

This patient calmed down rapidly and was able to cooperate fully with my examination. The temporary "cure" seemed magical, yet it occurred predictably after the patient identified, expressed, and had me understand the main potential danger for him—that of being humiliated.

After my examination, I felt I could supply him with the kinds of help he had originally requested and referred him back to his psychiatrist, feeling the transaction was complete and successful.

To use this approach most effectively, you must be willing to receive and understand the patient's point of view, including the *gravity and intensity he experiences.* You need not experience the actual fear the patient experiences, but certainly he must know that you understand the gravity behind his fear.

Communication and Purposeful Action

COMMUNICATION IS GIVING AND RECEIVING INFORMATION. This process is so basic to our everyday experience that a discussion of communication between individuals may at first glance seem superfluous. We are, after all, perfect communicators. We are marvelously equipped to get and give information. Our difficulties in communicating arise when we do not use our equipment to maximum advantage or when we do not appreciate the essentials of communication.

What are those essentials?

(1) Obtaining and giving attention.
(2) Clear communication delivery.
(3) Acknowledgement.

Attention is basic to any communication. You cannot talk effectively to someone who is not listening. It does no good to write a memo that goes unread. Attempting to communicate without first obtaining attention is the cause of dozens of daily irritations and frustrations. Many of these instances are trivial, to be sure, but failure to get and give attention as a first step to communication in health care can be a matter of life and death.

One trivial example: Your wife is reading a magazine when you suggest going to the movies that night. She says "hm-m-m," and continues reading. You are not sure you got her attention before beginning the communication, and you wonder whether you will ever get to the movies.

Another trivial example: You are at your desk, planning a Mexican vacation that will begin in two weeks, daydreaming about fiestas and golden Acapulco sunsets. A technician, passing your desk, says something. You have no idea *what* he said because he did not first get your attention. You have no choice except to stop him and ask, perhaps sheepishly, "I'm sorry, what did you say?"

In an emergency situation or in a health care situation with time limitations, the initial step of getting and giving attention, although essential to communication, often is overlooked. Persistence may be required to get the attention of certain patients focused on your communications. Hurried or worried patients often are distracted by the strange environment of the health care setting, by their physical condition, and by the reality shock caused by their worry. Yet, all attempts to get and give information are unsuccessful to the extent we fail to get and give attention.

Attention is equally essential in attempts to communicate with other members of the health care team. In a fast-moving dramatic situation, orders and other communications fly through the air. But is attention being given and received? Is anyone listening? Acting? Was attention directed to the air around the group, or to an actual person who could receive and give attention to the communication? In my experience I have found it effective to give and obtain attention to my communications in an emergency by using the name of the person for whom the communication is meant. "Joe." Yes?" "Hand me the. . ." "Mary." "Yes?" "Turn on the. . ."

Clear communication delivery, after giving and getting attention, is vital. The receiver must get an exact or close copy of what the sender has in mind to communicate. A mixed message may result when the words used actually have little or no relation to the intention of the sender. One woman may compliment another, for example, by saying: "What a *lovely* dress you're wearing." And it may be her intention to say just that. But if she says it in a voice that is sickeningly sweet and seems to be sarcastic, the same words reflect a different intention: "What a *lovely* dress you're wearing."

In health care situations we frequently receive mixed messages. One example would be the patient, obviously demanding attention, who says: "Leave me alone!"

We add nuance and gestures to words in the manufacture of a mixed message, which often is the truthful message.

We are perfect communication senders.

We are perfect communication receivers.

We get the whole message, even though we sometimes are reluctant to admit we get the whole message.

Communication is successful to the extent that it is clear, to the extent that the same picture or idea intended by the sender actually is received by the receiver.

But simple reception, no matter how clear, does not complete the communication. The communication cycle still has attention invested in it until the sender knows his communication has been received. Before the cycle is completed, the communication must be acknowledged.

Acknowledgement can take any form. It can be verbal: "Yes, sir." "Okay." "Fine." "I got it." It can be an action: a nod or actually carrying out the order immediately. The latter, however, assumes the receiver is visible, which often is not the case.

To test the importance of acknowledgement in the communication cycle, try an experiment. The next time you are talking on the telephone, receive all the communication from the other end and say nothing. Listen for the reaction.

To the extent a communiation is not ended with an acknowledgement, attention still is invested in the communication. Lacking acknowledgement, one of two questions is inevitable: "I wonder if she understood it?" or "I wonder if she understood that I understood?"

Unacknowledged, unended communications result in confusion and disperson of attention. It is good practice to complete each communication, ending each as it occurs. This fully frees attention for the next communication or for the next health care transaction.

How Patients Hear Things

JUST COMMUNICATING IN YOUR NORMAL EVERYDAY WAY TO patients most times isn't enough to really get the message across, unless you are one of those genuine down home types and very patient yourself. Otherwise, chances are that your normal everyday way of communicating has changed through your training and practice to become much more technical and, even more impacting in this situation, much more abbreviated. Not only that, the lay public has nearly limitless access to more and more accurate health and disease information, but still can at best be only partially learned, since these people are not practicing, expanding, and using the information as the health professional is.

For instance, when you are reporting to the patient the information that her pap smear is positive, count on that patient to hear nothing accurately beyond the word "cancer," or "carcinoma," or "possible growth process," or "abnormal cells." Having such heavy previous media exposure to "cancer" and all its semantic disguises, your patient likely is too busy *drawing conclusions* and *adding ideas* to really listen from that point on, no matter how accurately reassuring you as the reporter are being. Unless, that is, you, as the reporter of the information, are aware of this process and know how to compensate.

My dad used to say a particular saying to me over and over again as I was growing up at home. For year upon year my amused reaction would always be, "There he goes again." He would go around the house saying "repetition, repetition, repetition," then point to his forehead, think for a second and break up laughing, as if he'd just discovered the wheel. Occasionally he'd turn to me, at times I guess when I looked particularly dull, and say, "Ark, that's the secret of being understood: repetition, repetition, repetition." And then he'd break up again, the wheel once again discovered and shared.

You want to know about the part of the mind that

automatically *draws conclusions*, regardless of the amount of ac-curate objective information that is assimilated, and *adds ideas* in inverse proportion to the amount of assimilated objective informa-tion, ideas based on fears and internalized (and therefore ubi-quitous) momentary sources of danger.

Fears, of course, are apt to be strongest when they revolve around a person's own body, particularly since the cultural consensus is that one's body represents his only means of survival and participation. Not only are these fears the strongest, they are the most ubiquitous, erring on the logical side of too many rather than too few. Except that in these cases the mind errs on the side of many, many, too many fears for the perception process to work ef-fectively, and almost certainly in fact too many fears for actual op-timum survival itself. But our stated concern here is for that part of the survival process that we call listening or hearing or otherwise collecting information from the environment that helps in physical or bodily survival.

In the example above, then, the patient who doesn't optimally collect all available objective information regard-ing "cancer," a genuine potential life threat, is not optimizing her mental and physical response to a real condition. Or, just as unhealthy, the patient is so blocked after the idea of "life or well-being threat" is assimilated that she doesn't assimilate the informa-tion that the chances of any threat at all are finite and can be abso-lutely ruled in or out by an additional procedure. In the case where that additional information is not assimilated further, totally unwar-ranted fears of "not knowing" and "not knowing whether you will know" are added to the already accumulating layers. That is generally applicable when your verbal *and your nonverbal* com-munications, weighted because of your position in the patient's mind, report or hint at life or well-being consequences for the pa-tient. In the particular example above, the second most powerful fear, the fear of ending one's potential reproductive capacity, is also added into the formula.

In communication situations like these it is the health professional's responsibility to make sure, regardless of the circumstances, that the patient received your message completely, pretty much exactly as you meant it. Your three most powerful tools here are i) patience and repetition, ii) communications bridges, and iii) setting up a clearly understood open line of communication back to you, a line that does not invite embarrassment or a sense of scar-city.

Communications bridges are used to span a gap. A bridge gives the receiver some idea of what is coming and elicits willingness for that to happen. Suppose someone is talking to you and you feel you need to interrupt that person in order to clarify a misconception on which his or her communication to you seems to be built. There is an anticipated gap there: one minute the person is talking along, and the next he is getting interrupted. Rather than abruptly stopping the person you might say, "Excuse me, can I interrupt for a second?" That's a lot smoother, or more tactful, than, "Now wait a second, buddy." Using the bridge, you have spanned an anticipated gap and elicited willingness. That makes for better cooperation and mutual success. The same principle applies to our example above. One minute the patient is about to receive information about a rather routine examination and the next she is receiving news that you know has the potential to create great impeding fears, justified or not. You might span that gap by saying, "The results of this test dictate that we do another test to make absolutely sure that area of your body is healthy. There is no need for alarm. I doubt that anything will come of it, but it is very important for prevention that we rule out any possibility that you have or are developing a condition that needs treatment." Then go on, being quite direct. Remember that indirect hints or conspicuously avoided words invite more fears. After the bridge has been built and understood, express directly and repeat frequently key information and realistic assurances when those are appropriate. You may need to actively elicit response and questions. Then suggest and formulate together a plan to eliminate the doubt about the condition. Toward the end of the interview say something like, "My goal here is to have you leave this conversation with no unanswered questions at all. Do you have any lingering doubts about what is happening, what we plan, or anything else?" Be unhurried. Remember that your goal is to have the patient *have all her questions answered* or to know how she can get them answered and participate in a plan of action to achieve that.

After all immediate questions are satisfactorily dealt with, it is useful in some circumstances to pause in the interview, even physically to leave the room yourself for a few minutes, leaving the patient with a pad and pen to jot down any additional questions she may find in her mind or in discussion with an accompanying friend. Having created that opportunity for thought and for safety, return and deal with these immediate residual questions and concerns.

When that interaction is complete, be sure to establish that open line of communication back to you. This patient will be talking with close relatives and friends, and incomplete anecdotal information abounds about almost any condition or potential condition of the human body. Thinking alone, as the patient will do also, reinvites the doubts and questions, worries that are harmful to healthy and ill alike.

You want to remember as well that in order to

learn to practice health care in almost any capacity you had to learn a new language. That language is filled with jargon, abbreviations, foreign language fragments, and technology. Words that have become everyday usages among you and your colleagues are usually partly or wholly nonsense to the average patient. Assuming that the patient will ask or clarify is almost always a mistake. People are often so embarrassed to stop you and ask, thereby admitting ignorance, that they will go away from a conversation completely mystified, worried, and unhappy rather than ask you. Therefore you, as the possessor and purveyor of the information must take on the responsibility of eliminating this unnecessary mystery if you want to assure the desired result of as much patient certainty as possible given the real situation.

I once knew a patient who had been receiving treatment, often dramatic, for cancer. Six months into this highly intelligent person's nearly continuous therapy she finally got around to asking the physician why "carcinoma" was worse than "cancer." That mystery was perhaps minor compared to more major uncertainties, but nevertheless that question was "bugging" the patient beyond what anyone but her could have guessed. One day soon, I believe, it will be established beyond anyone's doubt that this kind of mystery and stress is a major component to all disease except perhaps the normal aging process. There is much the health care worker can do in informing the patient of the importance of certainty, within our present limitations, and affecting elimination of unnecessary mystery.

In a way you as the health care worker are "on stage" with patients. Right or wrong, patients have learned to give tremendous weight to what you say just because you seem to the patient to be more knowledgeable about, and therefore in more control of, a condition which leaves the patient feeling to some degree out of control. That is true to some extent whether your are the attending physician or the ward clerk. While you want to be warm and avoid robot-like posturing, at the same time you need to be aware of your nonverbal communications, remembering that your gestures are being given undue weight by many patients.

Listen to the Patient

At the same time you want to remain aware of the patient's nonverbal communications to you. Watch for sudden changes in the patient's countenance as you deliver information, opinions, doubts, or suggestions for action. A sudden dart of the eyes, jerk of the shoulder, or lessening of the patient's facial effusion at a point in the conversation when you are not delivering bad news may well indicate an unspoken question, a premature conclusion, or an added negative idea on the patient's part. Here it is appropriate to stop your conversation and do the one thing you can to find out: ask the patient.

"Listen to the patient. He is telling you what is wrong with him." How many times in your training or practice have people told you that? How many times has it actually been true in your own experience? Of those times when it really was true, how much of it did you see as soon as the information could have helped and how much of it did you see partly in retrospect?

The idea, of course, is to receive the whole gift of information from the patient as much as possible while it is being delivered, even when it is sent in pieces. The next best is to see it right while you are leaving the patient's side, when you can resume the conversation to complete your understanding of what the patient is telling you is wrong with him. It is never too late, providing you still have the patient, but it is best to have a very complete understanding of the patient's perceptions and ideas, and sometimes conclusions about, just what it is that is wrong. That understanding on your part is in itself worth as much as your knowledge and skill and all the finest technology that will ever be invented and in fact that understanding is requisite to maximizing the probability that you, as part of the care provider team, are doing the very best things you can.

Because patients are prone to adding ideas and drawing conclusions, you will want to elicit these and help the patient understand them and neutralize them. That elicitation requires a lot of patience on your part. Sitting through and actually remaining actively interested in the patient's conclusions can be very difficult, especially if they are delivered first, forcibly, fearfully, or doggedly. Because these conclusions are usually salted with fear, of an unknown or known but not completely identified danger, they often come across packaged with force, insistence, fear itself, blame, or something that looks like hostility. Nevertheless, it is all vital information, provided we know how to receive it without adding anything of our own.

Physicians As Communicators

Many, many times I have heard from patients, potential patients, and members of health care teams that physicians particularly are difficult to communicate with. With some extremely laudable exceptions, this observation is generally true for many people. When that problem exists, it is always a two-party problem. Physicians in our culture are widely seen as having the power of healing, possessors of mysterious knowledge, users of technology sophisticated beyond common understanding, holders of life and of death. It is absolutely not accurate that physicians hold the power of healing, but nevertheless it is a belief widely held because of its apparent convenience. It is clear to me at least that the only person who has the potential power of healing is the patient himself, and the physician and others on the health care team have the power to help the patient actualize or catalyze his own ability to heal. Yet the belief about physicians persists, and one's own power to heal, with appropriate and often vital help, is mentally and automatically assigned to the physician as symbol.

This automatic assignment of power has two driving forces behind it. First, it can seem to be an awesome responsibility to a patient. After all, thinks the patient, if I am responsible for the cure, then I am to blame for the condition. While that logic is spurious, and harmful, nevertheless many people fall prey to it. The physician then becomes exalted in the patient's eyes, and incidentally becomes the person to blame for the failures or slower than expected successes. The physician's part in creating his or her relative communication isolation occurs when the physician tacitly or overtly agrees to be placed on this exalted pedestal. Tacit agreement occurs when the physician develops and unconsciously manifests an image that amounts for others to relative unapproachability. If, for instance, the physician automatically projects a "very busy" image, people sense that and conclude, just as automatically, that this physician is "too busy for a little problem." This conveniently reinforces these peoples' own fears about communicating to such a "powerful" person. The result can be that the physician does not hear about some growing problems until they are "big enough to warrant his attention." Such automatic projections of "busy-ness" are quite distinct from actually being very busy but at the same time showing full unhurried attention and active interest in communication events themselves.

Physicians too are tempted to develop an "all-knowing" image, thus allowing for the "magic" curing effect on some patients. But when this image becomes automatic in its projection, then people around this physician are at times tempted to withhold potentially helpful information or alternative suggestions because this input doesn't seem needed.

Physicians who always seem stern and unbending run the risk of people supplying information or requests which they think will obtain approval, sometimes at the expense of accuracy.

And so it goes. Physicians, by their position, their projected images, and sometimes by their training, are often at a disadvantage in obtaining volunteered vital information. Physicians who are not falling into these traps themselves still inherit the problem through people's personal history of mistrust and awe with other physicians. Physicians, in their own and in their patients' interests, must often compensate by i) displaying full unhurried active interest, known as patience, ii) actively eliciting information, iii) projecting human fallibility or real doubt when that is appropriate, and iv) explaining fully his or her thinking, conclusions, projected plans of action, and openness to adjustment given new information or changes during the course of applying the plans of action. Physicians, other health care team members, and patients often benefit together when the physician as designated leader genuinely and repeatedly asks for help in the form of full direct communication among all participants in the health care interaction.

The Leader:
Master of Time, Stress,
and Confusion

STRESS IS AN UNNECESSARY ELEMENT IN GENERAL, AND IN particular, for our purposes here, is unnecessary in health care situations. Stress reflects the absence of knowing control, the absence of a clear sense that someone is willing and able to lead.

Stress is made up of confusion, time, and assigned importance. Because stress plays such a large and largely unnecessary role in so many health care situations, it is worthwhile to consider each of its ingredients in some detail.

Confusion is the dispersal of attention, the opposite of concentration. Confusion consists of randomness and results when we are expected or expect ourselves to do more than one thing at the same time. Confusion is an element in every crisis situation. Many incomplete problem cycles compete in order to reach the goal in each given situation. What are the most important problems? Where should we start? Who should do what?

Confusion seldom exists if the situation is familiar. The protocol is clearly established by past experience. There is no problem. A successful outcome will depend on the effectiveness of the protocol and the team's ability to alter or drop the protocol if it is not appropriate to the present circumstances.

The key to handling confusion in less familiar situations is to resist the temptation to try to *figure out* exactly what to do first. This usually results in hesitation and rarely results in efficiency. What works in a confusion situation, I have found, is to *begin.* Jump in, no matter where. Do one action; take one step. Taking one action in the physical world, no matter how brief or simple, begins a process of stabilization.

Example: In dealing with a multiply injured patient, I routinely feel first for the patient's radial pulse with one hand and palpate the neck with the other. This first action stabilizes my attempt to rapidly assess a potentially confusing situation.

The next step comes automatically. I examine; I '

see what's there. This leads to perceptions, the unevaluated impressions coming through the senses which I consciously list. When all perceptions are gathered, I begin making evaluations by fitting the perceptions into possible patterns. Making most perceptions first, before making evaluations, avoids the danger of jumping to conclusions. And taking that first step to stabilize the situation—doing something, no matter what—tends to eliminate confusion before it starts and becomes a potentially consuming matter.

Another ingredient of stress is time. When we are in a hurry to bring order to a potentially confusing situation, the two elements, time and confusion, weigh against each other. Getting it done quickly can seem to conflict with completely handling each of several problem cycles.

Time is an invention of people. It is an arbitrary measurement between events. There is not time without action or events. Time begins when a cycle of action starts. So *starting* an action—doing something, no matter what—positively affects two of the elements of stress. It not only helps stabilize confusion, it also helps regulate the time factor.

Importance is the third element of stress. Importance is a value assigned by people. Most people in our culture agree that preservation of human life is important. This value or importance is one of the foundations of health care in the United States.

An example of stress: A locomotive is steaming down the track, straight at your back. You turn as the brakes screech and the whistle shrieks with the locomotive just a few yards off. This situation has the elements of confusion, time, and importance.

What to do? At the instant of stress, we are reminded of all similar moments in our past, both experienced personally and observed in the experience of others. The memory offers a logical solution to the present problem: Jump. But the memory also recalls a similar situation in which jumping would have meant hurtling off a 200-foot trestle. So jumping may not be a usable solution now, and the mind instantly computes a conflict in solutions. The conflict compounds stress.

In a hurried health care situation, for instance, when handling certain types of emergencies, most of us are reminded of other emergencies, both personally experienced and observed in the experience of others. We are dealing with the emergency at hand under a certain amount of stress that is unnecessary.

We are reminded of similar cases we handled or saw handled with outcomes we considered failures. We are also reminded of cases that had one or two similar elements, but in the total view were completely different. Our initial reaction in these instances may be to begin to apply solutions that worked with the remembered emergency but which will not work in this instance.

We carry our own stress into these situations, and this hampers us in objectively viewing the elements of the present situation.

Our stress in hurried health care situations can be controlled if we realize that the emergency is the patient's emergency. The danger is his. We are there, participating, by choice. We can best serve the patient by being willing to take his point of view, but at the same time resisting the temptation to identify with his problem. By taking an action, we can control importance. By realizing that we ourselves are not actually in danger, we can preserve our objectivity and deliver far better care.

Leadership

A point is reached in the handling of every emergency when each team member has (1) felt initially confused and experienced a gut-level reaction, (2) begun to participate by taking one action, whether or not assigned, (3) made perceptions, and (4) evaluated the perceptions to form the beginning of an impression and individual plan of action.

From this point on, the situation will rapidly be stabilized, or it will rapidly deteriorate. It is at this point that every member of the team feels the need for assertive leadership.

Leadership cannot be established without communication. The first step in communication is to get attention. The leader or leaders must get the attention of the group at this critical point, a major turning point in the handling of confusion.

The leader gives orders, addressed individually to team members by name and repeated until the order is received and acknowledged by a nod or a verbal remark. The leader gives his assessment of the situation and outlines the general plan of action. This communication should be delivered decisively. It takes only seconds, yet it lets all team members know where things are going and gives each an opportunity to supply *appropriate* help.

Leadership must be accepted by the team members as well as assumed by the leader. This is an area of tremendous potential conflict. Without this acceptance, the forming team will deteriorate into opponency, factions, and ineffectiveness. Once leadership is assumed and accepted and the overall team plan is announced, the group offering care has become a real team, traveling in the same direction for the same purpose, rather than a group of individuals attempting to effect scattered individual plans.

Priorities become obvious. Delegation of responsibility is effortless. Team members know exactly what is needed by both the leader and the patient, and they can supply these things. Confidence emerges.

It is my experience that any harried situation, no matter how confusing initially, can be predictably stabilized and brought to conclusion using this general approach. This assumes competence and skill on the parts of all team members. But competence and skill, in my experience, rarely constitute a problem as serious as an ineffectual leader and team members failing to overcome stress and confusion. This general approach, I have found, is predictably satisfactory in solving this problem.

Children in Health Care

DEALING WITH CHILDREN IN HEALTH CARE, FOR MANY OF US, sometimes becomes an uncomfortable and frustrating experience. I think it is important to examine some of the common causes for these frustrations and to consider practical guidelines for handling both the young patient and their parents in health care situations.

One reason for our common frustration stems from the assumption that we, as adults, are somehow wiser than children and that we automatically know what is best for children in any and all situations. Adults certainly have more experience than children, but pragmatic experience does not necessarily lead to insight, and perception often is blinded by assumption.

Our adult picture of "what is best" for youngsters often is formed with reference to all children as a group rather than with reference to a particular child in a particular circumstance. We tend to assume that what works in one case with children will work in all similar cases.

In the health care transaction, we sometimes treat a child not as a responsible person who is our teammate, but as someone who must be talked down to, who is especially vulnerable. This may result from our own feeling that an injured or sick child is somehow *more* injured or sick than an adult with the same condition. In other words, we sometimes deal with children from a position of evaluation before perception. Often a pre-occupation with "what is best" for the child acts as a barrier to actually perceiving a particular child's situation. Just as we cannot see what the adult patient is experiencing if we prejudge what is best for him, neither can we comprehend the child's experience if we try to understand his needs according to some general rule. When we act on this basis, we are more likely to encourage balkiness or uncooperativeness in a child rather than calming the child and securing his cooperation.

A child, of course, is a person. A child is a person

of few years with a small body. A child is gaining experience of life and the world he lives in.

As a child goes through life, he constantly is looking for what will *work* for him in each situation to achieve the result he wants. As each new challenge or problem is solved, *the child acquires another remembered solution.* When a child encounters a new problem in the world, he looks for a solution. If the problem seems familiar, he draws on solutions that have worked in his past.

Watch a small child learning to perform a physical task: how to walk; how to tie a shoe; how to draw. The child will try over and over until he masters the desired skill. No matter how often a toddler falls in his attempt to learn to walk, regardless of any frustration he may feel, he gets up again and again, until, at last, he knows how to walk.

Learning in the physical world is exciting and rewarding for a child because *the ground rules are predictable.* In all the child's experiences, gravity does not change. The child soon learns that if an interaction with gravity is dramatically different from previous interactions, the difference can be accounted for in his own actions or in the situation. Gravity as a working ground rule is stable and predictable.

With people and situations, the rules and behavior are frequently less predictable. Nevertheless, the child's inclination is to proceed with the same learning steps he has acquired in the physical world; he persists in trying to figure out the problem and then find something that works toward its solution.

Even before we see a child in the health care setting, he has some "solutions" to the situation as he sees it. These solutions may or may not actually work in that situation. The most common types of "solutions" I have encountered in these situations are: (1) pretend the situation doesn't exist; nothing is wrong (the case of the disappearing earache); or (2) get out of the situation (try to escape by having to go to the bathroom in the middle of the procedure); or (3) fight the situation and everyone involved in it (the case of the screaming laceration patient).

We must remember that a lot already has happened to the child before we see him. The child's experience before we see him must be taken into account as part of our interaction with the child and his parents. Remember: *this child already has a collection of solutions tried and proven in many situations.*

The child's previous experience includes his experience to date with his illness or injury. A child's experience of an illness or injury event is similar to anyone else's. He senses mystery, identified or unidentified potential dangers, probable pain, and reality shock.

In addition, the child's experience before we see

him usually includes what he has been told, directly or indirectly, concerning this situation. Beyond his own experience, he has learned about the problem from his parents, grandparents, or the babysitter. If the parent senses great danger, appropriately or not, *this fear will be communicated completely to the child,* even if the parents do not actually say a word about it to the child. The child may be prone to use incomplete or conflicting information to form a belief about his condition or its consequences. Even though this belief may be inaccurate, *it often seems more comfortable and certain than the mystery resulting from incomplete information.* To the extent the child is in the habit of assuming his parents' point of view as his own, he will have this added factor, positive or negative, with which to deal.

For example, a child with a simple facial laceration may be wondering what will happen, but otherwise not be too concerned. If, however, the mother is very concerned about the danger of a potential scar, for instance, her sense of danger will be communicated to the child. If the child identifies with his mother's point of view, he will experience potential danger and fear. The child may know nothing about scars, or may not care, yet he senses some potential danger and adopts it as his own. The difference is that unless the mother has directly communicated with the child concerning scars, the child senses a completely *unidentified* potential danger, and the situation may seem much worse to the child.

This is the situation we frequently inherit. We have a child hurt or ill, who experiences a fear of potential danger— whether his own, or a parent's that he has taken as his own, or both—and who has experienced a sudden change in reality, or reality shock. In addition, his experience of health care may be limited, resulting in a wonder which will become worry. Or he may have had bad health care experiences in the past, bringing him to this situation with operating "solutions" of caution, fear, mistrust, or open panic.

I generally approach this situation in this way: I walk up to the child and address him *first and directly.* No matter what ideas the child or the parents may have, after all, this problem is primarily the child's problem.

Then I introduce myself briefly to the parents and explain that I would appreciate their help in letting me get most of the information I need directly from the child, without interruption. This gives the parents a way to help both me and the child and keeps them involved but not interfering.

In a friendly manner, I then turn back to the child, tell him my name, and explain where he is in terms of setting and that I am the doctor who will take care of him. I ask his or her name and address the child by his first name from then on. I make eye contact with the child and make a point of noticing what there is about this particular child at this particular time that is individual. If the child is over two, I offer my hand to shake and explain that I like to shake hands. If the patient is an infant, I ask the mother to continue holding the baby throughout the history and examination. If the child is screaming or upset or unwilling to answer me or give his name, I tell him I will come back in a few minutes or when he can answer me.

I ask the child if I can see where he's hurt, examine this and other necessary areas, and ask the child about what happened. Reviewing the illness or injury events may result in temporary upset but ultimately results in greatly increased cooperation from the child.

Then I seek the child's active participation in the health care transaction. In case of a laceration, for example, I explain to the child that stitches are needed to help fix the cut. I explain that I will need his help and make sure he understands the word "help." I tell him I want to make a trade, that I want to make a bargain or deal with him, and I make sure he understands these words. If the child does not come up with a definition himself, I supply this one: A deal means I do something for you, and you do something for me, so we help each other. The purpose here is to elicit his willingness and cooperation. In my experience, this procedure almost always is successful. I then say: "There are two things I can do for you. I can put stitches in which will help your body fix the cut, and I also will tell you everything I am going to do before I do it, so you will know what is going to happen." I make sure the child understands both parts. Often the child will ask me what he can do for me as his part of the bargain. If not, I tell him: "you can hold very still." If the child asks whether it will hurt, I say there will be one part that hurts for a short time and that I will tell him when that part is coming. The rest will not hurt at all, I tell him, although he may feel pushing. If he is upset by this, I do not try to minimize it. I say I understand that he doesn't want to be hurt (I also use a Number 30 needle to inject the local anesthetic).

In my experience, it never works to lie to a child in this situation, no matter how temporarily convenient or easier it may seem to us as adults.

I completely and consistently fulfill my part of the bargain, beginning with an explanation of my gloves, which I show to the child ("these keep everything clean, they are so thin you can see my fingernails through them, see?") and continuing through every step of the procedure. During this procedure, I frequently remind the child to keep still if this reminder is needed.

I tell him when the injection is about to start, and I tell him when it is over and that the rest will not hurt. I do not say he won't feel it because he may feel pushing. I say it is okay to cry if he wants but to remember to stay still. At the end of the injection, I thank him for holding still and for helping me by keeping still and for helping me by keeping his bargain with me.

I remind him that having the stitches taken out will not hurt and that he won't need any shots for that. This eliminates any potential worry in the intervening days needed for healing.

In the case of much younger patients, it is possible to relate to the infant as well as the parent. Ask the parent to hold the infant throughout the history and examination. Learn the sex and name of the infant, and don't call a girl "him." In the case of all infants, explain to the parent what you are about to do.

For infants over six months or so, tell the infant what you are about to do. Even if they do not understand the words, my sense is that they do get your intention to be friendly. Remember to show the infant your instruments before you use them. Demonstrate their use on the parent, if he or she is willing. Examine the mother's ear, for example, in front of the 10-month-old infant.

And remember the cardinal rule in dealing with any child: *Tell the truth.*

Handling parents can be more of a problem than handling the child patient.

Parents, like their children, usually have ready "solutions" even before we see them. The most common types of parental solutions I've observed which do not work are: (1) to side with the child against the doctor (or other health care provider) or (2) to side with the doctor against the child. Neither of these "solutions" work because neither produces support for the child, for the health care team, or for the parent. Still, we must know how to deal with these very common "solutions."

Here is an example of a parent siding with the doctor against the child: The parent turns to his youngster and says, "The doctor will give you a shot if you don't behave."

Here are examples of parents who are so overcome with fear and sympathy for the child that they tend to side with the child against the doctor: the parent who insists on speaking for the child; the parent who asks at the beginning of the transaction, "Does he have to have a shot?"; the parent who winces when the nurse brings the needle or thermometer near the child; the parent who tells the child that "it won't hurt."

Most child patients, I am convinced, resent these unworkable "solutions" of their parents. Most of us have had the experience of seeing a child settle down immediately after the parent leaves the room. And that brings the question: When should parents be present?

I have a few general rules.

When dealing with infants under one year, I prefer to have the mother present and holding the child comfortably throughout the history and examination. The exception is a lumbar punction or in the case of a laceration when the parent prefers to be out of the room. A parent who is in the room when he or she doesn't really want to be is a problem for everyone.

For a child over eight, I usually prefer to have the parents out of the immediate area once a procedure has begun. This allows the child to be on.his own with his own problem and results in a very successful experience and transaction.

For intermediate age groups (two to eight years), I do not have a general rule. Each situation is individual. The guidelines I use are (1) the child's preference, given a choice, (2) the parent's preference, given a choice, and (3) my own sense of whether the parent is truly able to support the child in this situation. More often than not, the parent stays and gives support to both me and the child.

If a parent is going to stay, I carefully instruct him to (1) sit quietly, (2) support the child quietly—for instance, by holding the child's hand during the procedures, (3) not interrupt, (4) not say "it's almost over," (5) be willing to leave at any time if they become uncomfortable or if I request it.

On the average, I have found parents understand the kind of help I need and, therefore, know how to help me and know how to help their child. They become completely supportive and a major asset to me in my work.

Most situations can be handled in such a way that active parent participation is an asset to you and to the child.

Handling children and their parents can be a joy.

Physical Pain

PAIN IS AN UNPLEASANT SENSATION WHICH CAN BE LOCATED in some part of the body. It is caused by physical, emotional, or both physical and emotional illness or injury.

Pain is a warning of danger. It is an indication of interference with optimum bodily function.

Pressure is a sensation created by the application of continuous force. It differs from pain in degree. As pressure becomes more intense, it is identified by patients as pain.

Pain can be intensified by the sufferer's attitude toward it. Most people experiencing pain try to resist it or avoid it in the hope it will go away. Concentration on resisting pain gives it more attention, with the result that the pain intensifies. Pain also is intensified by worry. The sufferer realizes that pain is a warning of danger, and this gives the pain enough importance to become a source of worry. Will it go away? Will it get worse? What does it *mean?* Do I have appendicitis? Cancer?

Two kinds of resistance, then, can intensify pain: resistance to the sensation of pain itself and resistance to the danger and possible future unpleasantness of which the pain warns.

The emotional intensification of pain by either form of resistance or by worry can magnify the pain to the stage of acute suffering.

Pain begins as a sensation and occurs with the impingement of stimuli on a kind of physiological receiving system. The sensation becomes pain when "too much" stimulus impinges on the receiving system. The more rigid the receiving system, the less stimuli required to create pain. A stimulus impinged on a relatively rigid receiving system will be interpreted as much more painful than the same stimulus impinged on a relatively resilient receiving system. This phenomenon, in medicine, is referred to as the "pain threshold." Whether accurate or not, the theory of pain threshold gives us a constructive approach in dealing with a patient who has pain. We know that as a patient increases his willingness to experience pain, the pain will decrease. We can help the patient overcome or control pain by assisting him in adding resilience to his stimulus-receiving system.

Two methods can be used to reduce rigidity in the patient's receiving system and thus decrease his pain:

(1) We can help the patient identify and, thus alleviate, his sense of mystery, worry, and danger. The patient's sense of danger adds to the rigidity of the receiving system. He is worried about what the pain means, and to this extent the receiving system has added rigidity. By explaining the meaning of pain, we reduce his worried sense of anxiety, his feeling of potential danger, reducing his receiving system's rigidity, and, thus, reducing the sensation of pain.

(2) We can help the patient to experience the sensation of pain instead of resisting the experience. Resistance to pain adds rigidity to the receiving system.

Some of this approach already is being practiced in medicine and is currently being taught in medical and nursing schools. Some of it is not, but probably should be. This approach is not meant to substitute for any existing diagnostic tool. It is meant to help alleviate pain once its diagnostic usefulness is exhausted.

This is how I put this approach into practice:

I first ask whether there is pain or pressure. If either exists, I ask the patient to identify its precise location by pointing to the exact area with one finger.

Then I ask the patient to describe the location in words. He may reply, "two inches below my belly button and two inches to the right of center." He may change the location later, but the process adds to his perception of his ailment.

I then ask the patient to describe the type of pain or pressure. Is it sharp or dull? Does it feel like a knife? Pins? A weight? A vise? And at this point *I always ask the patient what he thinks could be causing this exact pain.* The purpose of this question is not to have the patient make a diagnosis. That remains my responsibility. The question is asked in order to give the patient a chance to unload his ideas about his experience of pain, including his deepest fears and anxieties. This reduces his sense of danger. I never reject silly or nonsensical answers out-of-hand but let him continue stripping away layers of fear. Sometime during the dialogue, the patient will identify for himself the one or two possibilities which he considers the greatest threats. This identification, of itself, discharges much of the emotion smothering the actual complaint. I often observe a positive change in the patient's attitude at this point.

During this recitation of the patient's ideas and fears, it is important to be an interested listener. Do not offer your own ideas yet. Make neither more nor less of the patient's pain or pressure than he makes of it himself. Do not say whether you consider it serious or insignificant. Simply receive the patient's experience for what it is, as he is telling it. Hear him out.

Once the exact location and description of the pain is obtained, I ask the patient to describe its shape as he sees it. Is it round or flat? A triangle? A sphere? Conical?

After the shape, I ask for the color of the sensation if it could have a color.

Then I ask for the size, in inches.

Then I inquire about the sensation's volume. If it could hold water, how much would it hold? A teaspoonful? A cupful?

All of these questions—most of the interview, in fact—are designed to increase the patient's experience of the pain, to help him face the reality of the experience, and thus reduce his rigidity. More often than not, the method results in a dramatic decrease in the patient's unpleasant sensation or complete disappearance of the pain.

Pain Medication

One of the major ways that medicine can help people, in my opinion, is to alleviate pain. Pain medication is a valuable tool available for this job, but the sensation and timing of its use is important.

Both patients and doctors frequently use pain medication to avoid the issue of pain rather than truly to alleviate pain. This can be well-intentioned and still not work toward actually solving the problem. All of us have seen the results of unnecessary drug dependence on a daily basis.

Pain is useful in diagnosis. Pain also may be a signal of emotional overlay on the part of the patient. Pain medication is most appropriate after the usefulness of the pain experience is exhausted.

Fallibility: Pretending to Know

ALL OF US IN THE HEALTH CARE FIELD ARE IN POSITIONS OF enormous responsibility. We must make decisions, on a day-to-day basis, which have major effects on the well-being of those we treat.

This responsibility is a reality for us who deliver health care, and it is a reality for our patients and the public. This shared reality has created a very firm agreement in our society concerning the power, the authority, and, too often, the supposed infallibility of our responsibility. The agreement results in very high expectations: both the expectations that the public has of health care and, in addition, expectations that we in health care have of ourselves.

This agreement in our society is based on the premise that we in health care know what we are doing.

Sometimes I think the public expects too much of us in health care. Sometimes I think we expect too much of ourselves. But both the public and our professional peers have the right to expect that we know what we are doing.

This powerful agreement between the public and medical people puts us very much on the spot. We find ourselves endowed with enormous responsibility and tremendous authority. We are in charge, and it sometimes is a matter of life and death. People expect much of us, often unrealistically. They sometimes expect miracles. They think we can do anything, handle any situation, deal with any kind of health problem. We are told this so often that some of us, sometimes, come to believe we *can* do anything.

Of course, we make mistakes. When we do, they are very visible to ourselves, to those we work with, and to the public. This high visibility is more apparent now in the health care industry than at any time in history.

This constantly puts us on the spot. Having entered into this agreement concerning our knowledge and responsibility, having accepted at least temporary authority and power, having our efforts sometimes embarrassingly visible, it can be very difficult for us to admit "I don't know what to do in this situation."

This predicament used to literally keep me awake nights when on duty or taking call. Instead of sleeping soundly during lulls on duty I used to imagine all kinds of cases which might be called in or arrive unexpectedly in my domain. Vague pictures came into my head of what might happen at any time—the very worst disasters, the most subtle emergencies. And in dealing with each hypothetical case during those long, sleepless nights, *I didn't know what to do.*

The night-thoughts became nightmares when carried over to the reality of day-to-day health care situations. I discovered that, despite my thorough training and experience, I was posing as an expert on everything. Any kind of case can arrive in one's sphere at any time, after all, and if you are alone on duty, it's you or nothing.

Not only did I notice that I was posing as an authority on everything that might show up in my domain, I also noticed that, in certain areas of my medical knowledge and skills, I was pretending to know things when I wasn't really certain. I was pretending to know because, as an agreed-upon absolute authority on everything concerning life-and-death matters, it was unsafe for me to admit to not knowing.

I since have shared these insights with many physicians and others in health care. And I have discovered a big secret: We are all doing it. The subtle anxiety you sometimes experience comes directly from this area.

Before we can stop pretending to know, we must understand the nature of knowledge. For our purposes here, knowledge can be divided into three groups:

(1) What we are certain we know and have mastered;
(2) What we are certain we do not know and have not mastered;
(3) What we aren't sure whether we know, or know well enough.

The first area is no problem. The question is: How do we expand it?

The second area also is no problem. We simply choose whether to learn some bit of knowledge from this category, thus moving it into the first area, or not learn it and avoid situations where we will need to know it. That is, specialize.

The third is the problem area. It is the area of least awareness. Here is where we begin pretending to know, where we pose. This creates tremendous wasted emotional energy which we burn in hiding our uncertainty so neither peers, patients, nor the public will *catch* us not knowing something we pose as knowing. This results in needless mistakes, delayed consultations, unusual gruffness with patients and personnel, decreased job satisfaction, and probably higher turnover in our health care teams.

In my initial experience with this insight, I became concerned suddenly about one area of my medical skill. The skill was a simple one: being able to rapidly intubate anyone at any time under any foreseeable condition.

The concern did not make sense because, at that time, I was highly trained and experienced in this skill. At least, I'd had no failures. Yet there was some uncertainty attached to this area that was draining part of my attention away from patients, even patients with "routine" problems. I began noticing that I was slightly distracted by this uncertainty even while wrapping a sprained ankle. Whether or not the uncertainty about what *might* happen was justified, it was affecting my ability to relate with patients and team members. While it didn't make sense, it clearly was interfering. This nagging and partly hidden distraction always was there.

I had a choice. I could deny the problem existed, which would have been denying my experience of it, or I could ignore the problem because it didn't make sense, or I could do whatever was necessary to rid myself of the uneasiness.

After some hesitation, which only served to augment the problem, I chose the latter. I trudged up to the operating room and requested some instruction on something I felt I already knew. It was embarrassing. Yet I immediately recognized the abundant cooperation and unspoken willingness to help. It took five minutes to handle the problem, and it hasn't recurred in the intervening years.

How can we stop pretending to know?

The first step is to know what you are pretending. Ask yourself the question "What am I pretending to know that I don't want to get caught not knowing?" Be specific. Make a list.

Pick the one from the list which has highest priority for you.

Then choose. Do you want not to learn it and avoid situations where you might need it? Do you want to ignore it and see what happens? Do you want to learn it?

If you choose to learn it, write down everything you would have to do to master it fully. Include reading, asking questions, practicing safely, everything. Then *do* all those things until you are certain you have mastered it.

Proceed down your list in this fashion until you have no lists left.

This simple exercise and follow-up can release attention from getting caught with egg on your face and free this attention and emotional energy for you and your patients to use constructively.

But caution: If you're only pretending to want to know how to do something, don't do it.

Ultimate Crisis

THE RESUSCITATION ATTEMPT, UNDER MOST CIRCUMSTAN-
ces, is an effort often complicated by stress. Stress, as you probably
have experienced, can impede an optimal result.

As a health care team leader and team member,
there are some simple methods you can use to lessen this stress
before, during, and after the resuscitation attempt.

Before

Some problems can be best handled before the emergency, before
the complicating factor of stress is introduced. The potential confusion and error that centers around the mystery most of us attach to
machines, for example, can be eliminated or contained *before* the
emergency arises.

Our health care settings abound with complicated
machines. New machines, frequently even more complicated, constantly are introduced as the gear of our settings are replaced and
updated. It simply does not work to *assume* who knows how to run
what equipment, and the time to discover that an individual lacks
certain skills with a machine is *before* the actual emergency.

Regular machine-oriented inservices, beginning
and ending with no assumptions about who knows what, are key ingredients to smooth operation during an actual emergency. It is
tempting to cut corners here, and it is done far too much. To
assume that the physician or head nurse actually knows every facet
of the operation of a monitor, for example, is unfair to the physician
or head nurse. Giving these people an opportunity to express not
knowing *before* the emergency allows them to avoid any pretense of
knowing while dealing with an actual emergency. This approach
provides an opportunity for expansion of knowledge without unnecessary and costly mistakes.

Machine and equipment inservices should consist of orientation, instruction, and, most important, having each person actually *touch and use* the machine involved. This ensures that ability with that machine extends beyond conceptual understanding and into real-life competence in the physical world, where it counts.

Complete orientation to the skills needed by each respective team member can be approached in the same manner.

During

Stress during an emergency will be reduced to the extent that we realize the emergency is the patient's, not ours. We are participating in the resolution of the emergency, not in the actual experience of the emergency. The dangers involved are not actually ours; they are the patient's. It is not the doctor or nurse or technician who may or may not soon be buried, depending on the outcome.

Since the emergency is not ours, we do not have to be in a state of emergency or panic while handling the patient's emergency. Calmness and efficiency are just as contagious as panic. Orders delivered before obtaining the receiver's attention will be lost. Orders delivered with certainty and intention (saying what you mean and meaning it) will be received and carred out with efficiency. Orders delivered with indecisive intention will be received with uncertainty and incompleteness. Orders delivered with more than appropriate force will be received with resistance. If they are carried out at all, they will be carried out with resistance and resentment, often resulting in "unexplained" errors. Orders delivered into thin air, instead of directly to an individual, will be received by no one, by everyone, or by some people—all indiscriminately and unpredictably. Unreceived or unacknowledged orders will create wonder, add confusion, and increase stress.

Team leaders who attempt to communicate an overall impression and plan without getting the full attention of the team are leaders in name only.

Team members who do not accept the offered leadership oppose the formation of a truly effective team.

All of this adds to the confusion, tension, and rush of the resuscitation attempt and diminishes the patient's chance for survival and well-being.

After

What happens after the resuscitation attempt, whether or not it was successful, is nearly as important to the long range team effectiveness as the action itself. Failure to resolve these stresses at this point leaves them floating as a potential complication for the next team effort.

Immediately after the action, as soon as the patient's emergency condition is resolved, is the time for communication and correction. Correction cannot occur, of course, until a result has been produced.

People, on the average, are sensitive about being corrected. And members of an emergency medical team, as people, are no different. People often feel that *they,* as persons, are being *reprimanded,* rather than having something they have *done corrected.* Reprimanding people works beautifully to produce defensiveness. It does not work at all to produce better results.

After each major emergency, I recommend that you take a few minutes to get the team together and look at results and corrections. Here are a few simple rules to increase success in doing this:

(1) Notice and acknowledge what result was produced—what worked. All corrections then begin with the understanding that a result actually got produced.
(2) Make it safe for people to have made mistakes. This allows people to see mistakes without getting clobbered for them. With this added openness, you will notice people's increased willingness to spot their own errors.
(3) Encourage all members of the team, no matter what status, to notice and point out anything you could be doing better.

A respiratory therapist, for instance, can give valuable suggestions or corrections even to an experienced emergency physician. Status, in this case, has no corner on insight. Much of my present practical knowledge in medicine has come directly from experienced non-physician personnel—nurses and technicians who've had the fortitude to make suggestions for improvement.

(4) When a mistake has been discovered and acknowledged, insist that those involved take the responsibility to learn what they need to learn to avoid that mistake in the future. Follow up on this, and acknowledge the increased ability when it is demonstrated.
(5) Encourage full participation in these short sessions, and make certain to notice and verbally appreciate the everyday routine skills that consistently produce the overall result.

In my experience, these all-important post-emergency sessions never have degenerated to an encounter between personalities. They are not personal, after all; we are not discussing the people involved, but their actions. I have found, on the other hand, that these sessions produce palpable patient-care results almost immediately and tend to unify the team by making it clearer that everyone is working for the same result—the well-being of the patient.

Death

DEATH IS SURROUNDED BY MYSTERY. THE SUBJECT IS fraught with unknowns.

Objective information available to us concerning death is quite limited. Our objective understanding of the meaning of death is limited.

We do know a few things about death. We know, for instance, that it is the end of survival as we know it. It ends the survival of a particular body.

There are many things about death that we do not know objectively. We do not know, for instance, exactly what happens to the being or soul, assuming such exists, after death of the body. All human cultures have tended to fill in gaps in objective information about death with assumptions, giving rise to the many belief systems surrounding the subject. These belief systems vary enormously from culture to culture and from person to person within each culture.

Individual reactions to death will vary with the mystery and beliefs held by each particular individual.

Death means loss.

Death is the end of the cycle of bodily life or survival. It represents absolute loss of that body as a means of survival.

If a person believes that the person *is* the body or that body *is* survival, that there is no soul or after-life, that person will experience absolute loss in the death of a friend or relative.

The objective loss is companionship. The friend or relative who has died no longer is an active companion in the physical world to those who have been around him during his life. This loss of companionship is expressed in grief or sadness.

When we experience death of a loved one, we are confronting our own ultimate aloneness. This subliminal reminder greatly intensifies the experience of loss.

When a loved one dies, we are reminded of other

losses. These may include loss of other love relationships, loss of the battle to preserve life, and ultimate loss of the battle to survive, particularly in cultures where death is not generally considered a natural part of the life cycle. We are reminded of other deaths, including our own.

Frequently, we experience death of a loved one as a betrayal of trust. We think that person *should* be present in our lives as an active companion. This experience of betrayal is unreasonable, yet very real to most of us. Because it seems unreasonable, people often feel guilty about having such thoughts. They tend to deny this experience of feeling betrayed. Once a person denies his own experience, whether reasonable or not, the unexpressed experience is stuck within the person and persists subliminally.

Grief is another common experience associated with death.

The experience of grief is handled variously by different individuals. Some avoid noticing its presence. Many notice its presence and resist its expression. Others notice it and experience or express it completely or incompletely.

Incomplete experience or expression of grief at another's death results in persistence of that grief in one form or another. Some of us in health care deal on a daily basis with people experiencing loss of a loved one's presence or worrying about that possibility. There are two common mistakes, in my view, in handling people experiencing the grief accompanying death.

One of these mistakes is to try to *force* expression of the grief. The other mistake is to try to *suppress* it. Both mistakes stem from an intention to help. Neither does help.

Trying to force expression usually comes from the intention to help a person "get it all out." Perhaps that would indeed be helpful. But it doesn't have to happen at once, for instance on hearing news of the death. An individual may prefer to wait until he or she is at home, surrounded by supportive family and friends or even entirely alone, before expressing grief. Perhaps the best way we can support this individual would be to help contact family members and friends.

Suppressing expression of grief is equally not helpful. Suppression often is accomplished inadvertently by interruptions, by brusqueness or avoidance on our part, by not supplying an appropriate or safe physical place for such expression, and by undue and often unnecessary use of "sedatives" which dull the experience and protract the grief reaction.

Allowing or even encouraging a person to express grief is support. *Forcing or suppressing* it is not.

In my experience, what works in handling reactions to death is to get out of the person's way and allow him to express whatever he wishes. This means providing a *safe place* with privacy and relative sound proofing. It means communicating directly and honestly, without force or unnecessary frills, the information that the patient is dead. If there is a group, talk directly to the person closest to the deceased. It means doing this at a time when you can give full attention and listen completely. It means letting the family members know they did what they could in the situation, by getting the patient to your team, and that you did what you could.

Toward the end of such an interview, I ask the family what else I can do to help. I supply the kind of help I can and tell them, openly and directly, when I cannot supply a particular kind of requested help. We usually can help by establishing communication lines with the priest, minister, or rabbi, other family members, and friends.

Death in your health care setting affects every member of your health care team.

Too often, staff members think they should be hardened to death. They think it is expected of them, in their professional positions, to be completely objective about it. This can result in staff members *pretending* to be unaffected, while actually they are really quite moved. They may feel it *unsafe* to express their real emotions, assuming that everyone expects them to have become adjusted to death long ago in their training and experience. This non-expression or incomplete expression causes the loss to persist, and persistence will affect the care of the next patients. Persistent loss accumulates and will add to the stress felt by your team members.

What works with staff people is not to force expression, but to allow it when there is something to express. Expression of my own reaction at the loss, be it sadness or irritation at myself or the situation, frequently breaks the ice and allows others to express themselves and, therefore, end the loss experience. It usually takes only seconds or minutes.

This method at first may seem embarrassing or theoretical or even "psychological." In my experience, however, it does work to produce better patient care.

Triage

TRIAGE IS THE ADMINISTRATIVE DIRECTION OF PATIENT problems into categorized priorities. It is a solution to potential overwhelming confusion. It requires a flow of problems and demands the establishment of priorities.

Triage cannot occur without a flow of some sort. A flow is movement from one point to another. Drops of water moving from point to point through a stream bed, for example, create a flow. Flow involves time. Seen from a stable point at streamside, the flow of water is measured in volume moving past that point per unit of time.

From a stable point in an emergency department, or busy office, the flow of patient problems can be measured by the number moving through the setting per unit of time. The flow of patient problems in your setting is divided by priorities, dealt with accordingly within the setting, and moved to a disposition outside the setting.

As a tool to avoid confusion, triage can be effective only when a team has been formed and leadership established. Without an effective team and established leadership, priorities cannot be formed and maintained.

A priority is something with precedence in time and importance. Priorities are choices made according to the importance, severity, or salvageability of the patient's problem. The importance is a value assigned by people and, hopefully, agreed upon mutually. In most patient care priority systems, maximum or optimum preservation of life and human well-being are the goals, and the degree of threat to these is a measure of the severity of the patient's problem.

When a large, unexpected flow of patient problems threatens to overtax the capacity and adaptibility of your setting, confusion results. Triage, always important, is essentially important when the incoming flow of patients is overwhelmingly larger than the outgoing flow. What works in this situation is to (1) slow down the incoming flow, perhaps by triage to other facilities, or (2) speed up the flow within your setting and thereby speed up the outflow from the setting. What definitely does not work in such situations is (1) to get upset, (2) to become confused, and (3) to hesitate while trying to decide the best way to begin handling the increased flow.

The flow of patients through your setting can be speeded both inside and outside your setting. More space can be allocated to patient care within the setting, and more personnel can be called in to help handle the suddenly increased patient flow. Outside the setting, follow-up doctors and all personnel connected with patient disposition can be alerted so that the flow of patient problems, after having been sped through your setting, can triage to the outside.

Within your setting, the flow of patient problems can be speeded by creating new problems of equal or greater magnitude.

People tend to fuss with little problems almost indefinitely unless they have something more important to do. This truth is reflected often in the boredom and relative inertia of a slow day. The way to get the little problem solved, and fast, is to find or produce a larger or more important problem. And this larger problem will disappear or be solved most efficiently if it is followed closely by an even larger or more important problem. This continual creation of bigger problems speeds the flow of the problems that previously existed.

Triage can save the day in a disaster situation when many patient problems present themselves at one time. Triage presumes the establishment of categorized priorities, so in case of a disaster suddenly taxing your facilities, personnel can direct the patient flow according to agreed upon standards of priority. We begin with our basic standard of optimizing the preservation of life and human well-being. Everything we do is based on achieving this ultimate result.

We can categorize priorities accordingly:

(1) *Partially Treat First* those patients with life-threatening but ultimately solvable problems. Treating them partially and first presumes available time, space, personnel, and equipment. The degree of treatment offered is enough to maximally stabilize the patient and minimally drain resources.

(2) *Completely Treat First* those patients with minor and solvable problems. Once treated, these patients can be added to the personnel available to handle other patient problems. In other words, they can help. If they are unwilling or unable to help in

the disaster, they can leave your setting and thus create more available space.

(3) *Treat Later* those patients with relatively minor problems which are not solved readily, given available resources.

(4) *Treat Last* those patients whose problems are non-solvable, given the available resources.

Other triage systems can be developed along the same basic principles to speed the flow of patient problems. The system outlined closely approaches our basic goal of optimally preserving human life and well-being.

The Anatomy of a Medical Emergency

THE PATTERN OF MOST LIVES IS PREDICTABLE, NORMAL, perhaps even humdrum and a bit boring. People are educated, go to work, or enter the professions. They marry and have children. They grow older and see their children and grandchildren through education and into careers, marriage, and parenthood.

This predictable pattern usually is enlivened by an occasional or frequent crisis, a situation which may change the normal course of events and which always demands a personal decision on the part of the individual directly involved. Crisis involves choice, permitting a person to make visible his own determination in life.

A man loses his job. This is a crisis, giving an opportunity for choice and decision. He may decide to pull up stakes, uproot his family, and try his luck in another part of the country. He might obtain work in a different industry where his talents would flourish, where he would become a real success. His children certainly would make new friends in a different environment, and they might develop along completely different lines. The crisis of losing a job, and the man's selective response to that crisis, could affect the evolution and growth direction of his family for generations to come.

A woman is in love with two men at the same time for different reasons. This is a crisis. She has a choice, and she can choose either the man who is happy-go-lucky, almost irresponsible, but always a lot of fun, or the steady, stable chap with a dry sense of humor whom she knows will be a good provider. She realizes her decision between the two will affect her life style and security. She may even decide not to decide, averting the crisis by waiting for another man who has all the attributes of these two. And this is the point: the decision which will resolve or avert the crisis is hers and hers alone.

Crisis always involves choice, the opportunity for

97

the person involved to make his own decision and the time to consider alternatives.

The medical emergency always involves choice, personal decision, and time.

A person's life is progressing more or less normally, perhaps with a crisis now and then to add spice. Then, suddenly and unexpectedly, totally without warning, he experiences a change in reality over which he apparently has no choice, no control, no time for deliberation or thought, no experience upon which to base personal decisions. He may be suffering physical pain or mental anguish. His very survival may be threatened. There is mystery; his future cannot be predicted. He may not know what is wrong. He probably does not know how it will be made right, or whether it can be. He is worried, distraught. The stakes are high. The dangers are real. And in this perilous moment of his life, he cannot take matters into his own hands; he cannot make his own decisions; he has apparently limited choice. He must depend on the knowledge and experience and compassionate interest of total strangers. This is the most dramatic of human situations. It is the medical emergency.

The star of this medical emergency drama is the patient. Always! It's his life, his pain, his suffering, his anxiety that make the drama. It may seem axiomatic to say this, but it is necessary because we in emergency care sometimes begin to think that *we* are the stars. The ambulance driver, seeing people turn to stare after him as he speeds through the streets with sirens screaming can sometimes think *he* is the star. Health care professionals sometimes think *they* are the stars. The only star of the real-life medical emergency is the patient.

But every star, as anyone in Hollywood can tell you, needs competent direction and excellent support from other players in the drama.

To provide happy endings for these real-life dramas, to avoid as many tragedies as possible, the director and each supporting member of the emergency care team must be superbly trained. Each must realize that the successful handling of medical emergencies requires three distinct abilities: (1) creation of meaningful communication; (2) utilization of technical and medical competence; and (3) control of confusion.

(1) In handling emergencies, we must be willing and able to make decisions, make things happen rapidly and accurately, and accept responsibility for the results. In order to add effectiveness to our own efforts, we must be able to create meaningful communication with those working with us—communication that causes prompt, accurate action on the emergency care team.

And we must be able to communicate effectively with the patient.

(2) Before dealing with emergencies, we must have estabished excellence in our competence and skills. Equally important, we must know when, where, and how to apply these skills. We must be selective. We must know which knowledge is useful and which is not, which experiences we can draw upon and which we cannot, what we can do, and what we cannot.

(3) We must know how to bring order to a confusing situation. There is a certain element of confusion in nearly all cases of emergency care, no matter how well-trained the team delivering that care. Confusion almost always exists in situations which seem to be new or overwhelming. To eliminate or, at least, stabilize confusion, we must be decisive. We must resist the temptation to hesitate, to deliberate at length on the best course of action. We must choose and begin.

To control confusion we also must have established certainty in our ability to direct flows of patients and patient problems. This ability can spell the difference between success and failure, especially when the work load is abruptly increased by the rapid arrival of patients during a local disaster.

Finally, we must accept responsibility for our decisions. We must be able to intercede responsibly, hopefully with grace and respect, in another person's life with decisions which almost certainly will change that person's condition, perhaps forever. This complete acceptance of responsibility for what we do and for the results obtained can, indeed, be tremendously gratifying.

Before we can accept this kind of responsibility to the patient, we must have developed a willingness, a desire, and a demonstrated ability to help. To truly help (to supply what is needed or wanted by another human without undue assumptions on our part) is basic to the success and joy in giving emergency medical care.

This, then, is The Anatomy Of A Medical Emergency. It involves unexpected danger, usually accompanied by pain and anxiety, for a person who suddenly finds himself a patient dependent on the decisions of others for his own well-being. It demands urgent action from a trained team capable of communicating, selectively applying acquired skills and knowledge, controlling confusion, and accepting responsibility, wanting to help.

Relationships:
Who Wants What?

A RELATIONSHIP INVOLVES SOME FORM OF CONNECTION. The simplest relationships involve a connection between two entities, whether between two people or only between separate parts of two persons or personalities. Two people may be totally committed to their relationship, in other words, or they may be related only in a specific area of interest.

People can have multiple relationships between themselves. Two men, for example, may have a business relationship, and at the same time they may be personal friends and competitors on the golf course. A man and woman may have one relationship as marriage partners and quite a different relationship as parents of the same children. One relationship between two people need not impinge on other relationships between the same two people.

Most relationships between two people involve a shared challenge, and a challenge presumes a problem. A problem is something we want changed, and the challenge is to change it. The problem could be a situation or condition in life that we want and don't have, or it could be something we have and don't want. The desire to change an existing situation, condition of life, or state of being is the beginning of the challenge.

The most successful relationships are those in which two parties agree to solve the same problem together by meeting the challenge in the same manner.

Example: A man and woman want to change their present sitaution of being single, friends, and lovers, to a state of being married and creating a family. This is the problem, and it is possible for the two to meet the challenge successfully.

Example: A physician and a recently hired nurse want to change their present situation of being strangers and become effective members of the health care team, working together. This is the problem, and it is possible for the two to meet the challenge successfully.

Relationships between two people usually begin with a basic intention, identification of the problem or desire for change, and an agreement to meet the challenge together. There is a shared problem and a shared willingness to meet the challenge. Such relationships *begin* successfully.

Frustrations in relationships usually are caused by secondary intentions hidden or unidentified from the beginning by one or both of the persons in the relationship. A secondary intention differs from the primary intention that is the basis of the relationship. It may not be in conflict with the primary intention, but it is different and added onto the primary intention.

Example: A man and woman want to change their present single status, marry and create a family. This, as before, is the problem and the challenge.

But the man, in addition, may have a secondary intention of sharing his wife's future inheritance. He may consider this secondary intention to be wrong, degrading, or deceptive. He thinks his wife, and certainly his father-in-law, might agree with this assessment. He decides he must hide this secondary intention from everyone concerned, including, eventually, himself. But the secondary intention does not go away; it simply goes out of sight.

The woman involved here also may have secondary intentions in meeting the challenge of marriage and family. She may desire marriage to this man to increase her own status in the community. Deciding that her secondary intention is hardly laudable, she may try to hide it from her husband. She must not, therefore, get caught *liking* the status that evolves from her marriage. If she gets caught liking this status, it may be discovered that her desire for it was one reason for marrying in the first place. She has to pretend that she does not like it and does not want it, blunting her own enjoyment. And if the husband enjoys contributing status to his wife, he is frustrated and confused.

Secondary intentions on both sides of the relationship thus can set the stage for frustration and drama.

Example: A physician and a new nurse want to change their situation as complete strangers to become effective members of a health care team.

Both, however, have secondary intentions.

The physician has discovered he is effective only in his sphere of health care operations. He has tried to become a community leader by running for both the Board of Education and the City Council, and in both instances he has failed. He feels ineffectual as both a husband and father. But in the health care setting he is so respected that he is tempted to swagger a little. He wants the active assistance of this new nurse for the support she can give to maintain or even improve his professional position.

The nurse readily agrees to the primary intention of this new relationship, the improved teamwork necessary to effective health care. But she has the secondary intention of resisting any threat to her personal individuality. Her intention to maintain her individuality, then, constitutes her secondary intention, and she is likely to interpret any overture on the part of the doctor as a danger to her secondary intention.

In these examples, the married couple, the doctor, and the nurse each had secondary intentions judged by themselves as being so inappropriate that they must be *hidden* from the other person in the relationship as well as from the person himself.

When in doubt about a secondary intention, communicate it directly to the other person at the beginning of a relationship or when you rediscover it. You may be surprised to find real acceptance and willingness to pursue the relationship.

In the absence of this communication and understanding, the long-range discomfort between the people involved will cause the relationship to numb. On verbalizing your secondary intentions, however, you may find they are truly unacceptable to the other person in the relationship. In this case, you can change your intentions, change your partner, or continue the relationship with the knowledge that there is an area of potential conflict and danger.

Once secondary intentions are communicated and either accepted by the other person or adjusted, the mutual joy of giving and receiving exactly what is wanted in the relationship can increase enormously.

INDEX

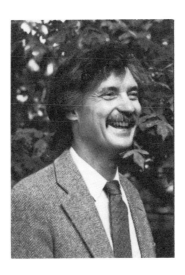

BIOGRAPHY

Arthur R. Ciancutti, M.D. likes to be called Arky. He was born and raised in New Kensington, Pennsylvania, near Pittsburgh. During his high school years he received a grant from the National Science Foundation to study at Bucknell University and at that point developed an interest in basic science. In 1965 he was graduated from Swarthmore College, where he studied chemistry and mathematics. During his college years, working from various private industry grants, he did basic medical research at Women's Medical College in Philadelphia. He received his M.D. degree from Case Western Reserve University School of Medicine. He did his residency in pediatrics at the University of California San Francisco Medical Center. During his early years in practice he became interested in the topics of trust, teamwork, and stress as they affected the causes of disease and the effectiveness of health care services. He practiced emergency medicine full time for seven years, partly as a means of studying stress and teamwork. In 1973 he formed the Natural Learning Center, Inc., an organization based in San Francisco, California, and devoted to research and practical training (*Dynamics of Teamwork*) in teamwork and stress-elimination for groups of people who work together and also for individuals. He has published widely in health care and business periodicals. Along with his writing and speaking, the Natural Learning Center is now his full time pursuit.

His hobby is the Brewery Gulch Inn, in Mendocino, Ca., a coastal farm which Arky converted to a bed and breakfast inn in 1983.

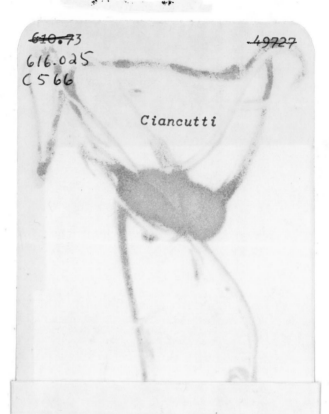

Ciancutti